MW00427502

THE PRICE
SHE PAYS

THE PRICE SHE PAYS

Confronting the Hidden Mental
Health Crisis in Women's Sports—
from the Schoolyard to the Stadium

KATIE STEELE, LMFT
AND
TIFFANY BROWN, PhD, LMFT
WITH ERIN STROUT

Little, Brown Spark
New York   Boston   London

Copyright © 2024 by Katie Steele and Tiffany Brown

Hachette Book Group supports the right to free expression and the value of copyright. The purpose of copyright is to encourage writers and artists to produce the creative works that enrich our culture.

The scanning, uploading, and distribution of this book without permission is a theft of the author's intellectual property. If you would like permission to use material from the book (other than for review purposes), please contact permissions@hbgusa.com. Thank you for your support of the author's rights.

Little, Brown Spark
Hachette Book Group
1290 Avenue of the Americas, New York, NY 10104
littlebrownspark.com

First Edition: June 2024

Little, Brown Spark is an imprint of Little, Brown and Company, a division of Hachette Book Group, Inc. The Little, Brown Spark name and logo are trademarks of Hachette Book Group, Inc.

The publisher is not responsible for websites (or their content) that are not owned by the publisher.

The Hachette Speakers Bureau provides a wide range of authors for speaking events. To find out more, go to hachettespeakersbureau.com or email HachetteSpeakers@hbgusa.com.

Little, Brown and Company books may be purchased in bulk for business, educational, or promotional use. For information, please contact your local bookseller or the Hachette Book Group Special Markets Department at special.markets@ hbgusa.com.

ISBN 978-0-316-56747-3

LCCN is available at the Library of Congress

1

LSC-MRQ

Printed in Canada

To my family. You are my lifeforce. I love you most.
—Katie

To my Grandma and Papa, your unconditional love gave me more than
I could ever explain. And to Tatum. The stronger the winds,
the stronger the trees—forever in awe of our strong roots.
—Tiffany

To athletes everywhere. You pay the ultimate price.
And we hope you always find your way back to yourselves.

CONTENTS

AUTHORS' NOTE

The Price She Pays relies heavily on telling the stories of real athletes who have coped with various mental health conditions. And for many, these conditions have intersected with their experiences of racial discrimination, colorism, misogyny, heterosexism, and gender bias. These women and girls share their deeply personal experiences, which include abuse, trauma, self-harm, substance use, mental health diagnoses, and suicidal thoughts. While some sources have agreed to be named, others have spoken on the condition of anonymity. For all cases in which a name has been changed, we mark the name with an asterisk on its first reference. To protect their confidentiality, we've also altered some dates, and minor identifying details have been changed.

Throughout the book we predominantly use the terms *girls* and *women*, but we know that gender exists on a spectrum. We honor the many ways that people feel connected to girlhood and womanhood. Currently, sports continue to operate on the binary with women's teams and men's teams. We know that stories about what it's like for athletes on the spectrum of gender are best told by people who share in this community and can give those stories the justice they deeply deserve. We included the anecdotes that we knew we could accurately tell, while recognizing the many ways that people experience women's sports. We look forward to seeing how sports can evolve to increase inclusion for all athletes, however they identify their gender. We also acknowledge that not all caregivers are parents—raising and supporting children is the job of many, whether it's grandparents, foster parents, other relatives, or guardians. We use the word *parents* throughout the book, but we know that the definition is vast.

We believe girls and women. We also believe that when they are empowered to tell their stories, it leads to systemic changes under which they train and compete. The stories you read in this book represent many identities across ethnicity, religion, race, financial status, sexual orientation, gender, gender expression, and identity. The stories within this book are verified through medical records, supporting documents, and/or corroborated by appropriate sources.

THE PRICE
SHE PAYS

INTRODUCTION

This all started in 2014 at a spin class. We'd find ourselves standing in that Eugene, Oregon, parking lot after each workout, talking about the heaviness we felt while working with athletes we'd been supporting as mental health professionals, mostly at the point when these young people were exiting their sports. Not only did they encounter difficulties in that big life transition but they also seemed to have so much left to process about their experiences. In our many conversations after spinning, distinct patterns about athlete mental health emerged—enough for us to know that we had a lot to explore when it came to systematic abuse, exploitation of athletes, racism, sexism, and more.

By the fall of 2021, Katie had started reexamining her own harrowing experience as an NCAA Division I track and field athlete, collecting medical documents from that chapter in her life, talking to former coaches and teammates, and writing down her own recollections. As we talked to more athletes over those years, we discovered that Katie's experience was, unfortunately, not so different from many others, across every level of competition. We believed that to start changing systems that clearly haven't supported the mental well-being of female athletes, we needed to tell the plethora of stories of those who have experienced them firsthand. Ten years in the making, this book is the result.

KATIE

From the start, sports have always been a means of connection for me. I cultivated my values, discussed worldviews, laughed, shared stories, and bonded with my dad during the many early morning miles we ran together. It deepened my relationship not only with him but also with myself. Living in Oregon, my favorite family ritual was our "peak of the week," when the four of us—my mom, dad, sister, and I—climbed nearby scenic mountain tops together. Exploring the outdoors became a natural part of my life, and I realized that movement alongside the people I loved just felt good. It became transformative.

Leading up to high school, I ran in community track meets and played soccer, volleyball, and basketball. But I *really* took to running. The summer before my senior year of high school, the phone rang, letters arrived, and coaches told me I'd have the opportunity to run at the university of my choice. College recruiting was on, and my passion was turning into opportunity before my eyes.

I have always been driven and highly motivated, so I was fortunate that during those formative years I was surrounded by family, coaches, and teammates who created a low-pressure environment. Fun and fulfillment were the priority, allowing me to progress at my own pace with a healthy connection to coaches who believed in me regardless of my results. Nobody could put more pressure on me than I had already placed on myself, and I always felt that they valued me as a human being, not merely as an athlete. That culture produced results, too: as a high school junior I placed in the top three in the state of Oregon in the fifteen hundred and three thousand meters. I went on to win the 2003 state cross-country title as a senior, too.

NCAA coaches visited our house. I visited campuses. I was offered full-ride scholarships. Then I made an early decision to attend the University of Oregon. My choice was based less on the iconic history of the track and field program and more on the reassuring presence of Marnie Mason Binney. She had been my coach during my freshman year of high school and moved on to the program at Oregon. I trusted her. She was familiar and understood my needs as a young, developing athlete. My connection to her felt real.

But when I arrived in Eugene, I found a program much different than what I thought I had signed up for. Teammates were pitted against each other, competing for rank. I sensed unspoken rules about food— what I was "allowed" to eat and when, and, of course, how much. Based on measurements and appearance, team members were told to lose weight but never given guidance on how to sustain our health; the priority was results. The camaraderie and community that had pulled me into the sport were replaced by tension, confusion, and mixed signals. My roommate, who was also my dear friend and teammate, and I were confused about a lot of things. What were our bodies supposed to look like? What was our place on the team? What were we supposed to eat? Was it normal to feel anxious when trainers and medical staff squeezed our backs, arms, and bellies with calipers to measure our body fat? By winter, several women were cut from the team, including my roommate, leaving me without the one person who felt like an ally.

Marnie resigned from her coaching position by the end of my first year. It wasn't until fifteen years later that she told me she found it impossible to coach with integrity in a program that fostered such a toxic culture. Her boss had watched her from the grandstands at Hayward Field and demanded that she "thin the herd of fat pigs" and "fat cows." At staff meetings, she said, he called athletes "cunts." Marnie documented the language and reported the behavior to the athletic director. More than a decade later, it finally made sense why the program I had entered seemed dramatically different than what I imagined it would be.

A new coaching staff arrived in Eugene in 2005, which unofficially included the now disgraced Alberto Salazar. He was involved in the program because his protégé, Galen Rupp, had been recruited to compete for the Ducks. We were all aware of the long-standing relationship between Galen and Alberto and assumed Alberto's presence was a condition of Galen's commitment. My new coach was Maurica Powell, then a twenty-four-year-old rookie who reported to head coach Vin Lananna, the man "responsible for creating a vision for the Oregon Track & Field program and Historic Hayward Field as the center of track and field in this country," according to the University of Oregon Athletics website.[1]

Many friends held Vin in high regard, and I was excited for the opportunity to train with him. But despite working hard to earn his praise and competing well that fall, the wheels came off at the end of the season. I asked my coaches for help, unable to find my fifth gear. In hindsight, I had all the symptoms of RED-S (relative energy deficiency in sport—a mismatch between caloric intake and the body's demand for nutrition, which can lead to amenorrhea and low bone density, resulting in injuries). I even told one coach I hadn't menstruated for months. The response? "That's great—your body fat is where we want it to be." It was, of course, unsustainable, and my performances began to falter. Unable or unwilling to recognize my struggle, my coaches told me not to come to practice until I was ready to compete again.

In some ways, the writing may have been on the wall when I decided to become an NCAA Division I athlete. I've always operated in overdrive. When I trained, I approached it with intensity. More was better, I thought. I was going to do whatever it took to perform, at any cost. The price, as it turns out, was quite high. Now I understand that when these common traits of high-achieving athletes are nurtured with care, they can turn into big advantages on the field of play. When they're exploited, they can break you.

I internalized my problems, took responsibility for my failures, and felt that I wasn't living up to the standards I was recruited for—standards I knew I should have been able to achieve. By the spring of 2006, it was Alberto who approached me with a supposed solution, when I was most vulnerable. He referred me to Dr. Jeffrey Brown, a Houston-based endocrinologist who diagnosed me, at age twenty, with hypothyroidism, a condition that can lead to weight gain and fatigue.

Dr. Brown prescribed medication and gave me hope. The combination of a powerful, elite coach like Alberto and a medical professional offering support made me feel heard and seen.

However, I became prone to passing out. At the emergency room in Eugene, I was diagnosed with iatrogenic (doctor-induced) hyperthyroidism, a fact I didn't actually remember until I started investigating my medical history in 2021. The Oregon ER doctors and a local endocrinologist immediately took me off the medication and my thyroid function stabilized within two months. Shortly after, in a choice that confuses me to this day, I went back on the thyroid medication. Ultimately, I put my trust in Alberto and Dr. Brown. I felt they understood my medical needs as an athlete better than the medical professionals at the local hospital. But the medication did nothing to help my performance. Hopeless, defeated, and exhausted, I quit the team with a couple of years of eligibility left. Alberto offered me a spot on his professional (now-defunct) squad, the Nike Oregon Project, but I declined. I wanted to finish college on an NCAA team, so Alberto helped me transfer to Florida State University.

I ended up in the new program with a coach who increased my mileage quickly. Even after I got injured, I was unable to back off on my own. With a stress fracture in my foot and torn tendons in my ankle, I went on to graduate as quickly as possible. Through it all, I remained connected to Alberto and Dr. Brown, who continued my treatment and collected my blood samples long after I had stopped competitive running. My now husband, Adam, who was an NCAA track and field champion and had spent five years as a professional track and field athlete, where he observed doping and corruption unfold on the world stage, found the arrangement suspicious. I wish I had, too. I have come to believe that I was a test subject in a larger experiment that they were conducting that involved using prescription medications (not banned by anti-doping agencies) to enhance athletic performance—altering my medication and tracking weight fluctuations to determine dosages that led to ideal metabolism and weight loss. Why else would a man who was no longer my coach have continued monitoring my bloodwork?

I was fortunate that my local Oregon endocrinologist kept comprehensive notes because when I began investigating my medical history in 2021, Dr. Brown's office stated that it had no records or documentation that I was ever his patient.

In 2015, the US Anti-Doping Agency (USADA) began investigating Alberto and Dr. Brown after several former Nike Oregon Project athletes and staff alleged that they were encouraged to take unprescribed medications, including thyroid drugs, to enhance performance. In 2019, USADA banned Alberto and Dr. Brown from the sport for four years for "orchestrating and facilitating prohibited doping conduct,"[2] though the charges didn't include the use of medication. Among Alberto's violations was possession and trafficking of testosterone (a banned substance), as well as tampering with the doping control process. Dr. Brown was charged with tampering with patient records, illegal administration of a supplement called L-carnitine, and complicity in trafficking testosterone. Despite the sanctions, Dr. Brown was able to retain his medical license and practice.

In 2019, Mary Cain, a former teen track star who trained professionally under Alberto from 2013 to 2015 at the Nike Oregon Project, came forward with her own story of abuse.[3] She said Alberto had weighed her in front of teammates, publicly body-shamed her, and offered her prescription thyroid medication to help her lose weight, after which Mary suffered depression, suicidal thoughts, five stress fractures, and didn't menstruate for three years. She sued Nike and Alberto for $20 million in 2021, alleging emotional and physical abuse. The lawsuit was settled in November 2023, but the terms of the settlement were undisclosed.

In July 2021, the US Center for SafeSport permanently banned Salazar from coaching USA Track & Field athletes based on charges of sexual misconduct. Kara Goucher, also a former member of the Nike

Oregon Project and a world championship silver medalist, later revealed in her memoir[4] that Alberto had sexually assaulted her during massages.

Each time another news story like these appeared over these years, it gave me pause and reflection. I wrote letters to authorities and others who might find my experiences and insight helpful—or add context to the memories I was piecing together. I never received replies, so my default response was to compartmentalize: to leave these experiences in the past and live my own life in the present.

In 2014, at age twenty-eight, my fertility doctor told me that I had been treated for a thyroid condition I never had, just as ER doctors had determined years before. I still take the thyroid medication because my body now relies on it to function. I take it every day and will need to keep taking it every day, for the rest of my life.

I still wrestle with the fact that I will never know if my health struggles are because of the "care" I received from Dr. Brown or not. But I do know that it took more than a decade for me to see the abuse I went through as an athlete for what it was.

Today, I'm a licensed marriage and family therapist, cofounder of Thrive Mental Health, an outpatient clinic in Bend, Oregon. I'm also the founder of Athletes Mental Health Foundation, a nonprofit organization designed to amplify athletes' stories and provide mental health resources for parents and coaches. But more than that, I'm a mother. Our three kids, Camden, Brooke, and Gavin, are my entire world. They are my core motivation to ensure sports serve as empowerment for youth and stoke a lifelong love of physical activity. I now know that I was called to this field specifically to help young female athletes, because that is what I needed at their age. I have a relentless desire to raise awareness and prevent unnecessary suffering for others by integrating mental health care into sports.

The more I've talked about my experience and processed what happened, the more I've realized much of what I went through as an NCAA athlete is not unique. In sharing my story and my expertise, my hope is that parents, athletes, and coaches can find support, advice, and hope for healthier, happier careers in whatever sport they choose, at whatever level they compete.

TIFFANY

My earliest connection to sports was forged over many hours spent sitting on my grandfather's lap, watching boxing matches, football games, and golf tournaments. Spending time with my Papa, who was a father figure to me, was all about sports. He loved teaching me about the games and the players, and I loved learning. I wanted to understand the rules and the strategy while spending as much time together as possible. Sports became the foundation of our close relationship as I grew up.

I remember watching Chi-Chi Rodriguez, winner of eight PGA events, whose charisma and love of the game captivated me—especially his trademark dance celebration every time he sank a putt. In retrospect, cheering for Papa's favorite athletes and teams helped me find my own passion for sports, although at the time, of course, they were all male-dominated. I had posters of Shaquille O'Neal on my bedroom walls, and I was a diehard fan of the Portland Trail Blazers. I don't ever remember turning on a game with female athletes when I was young, though it never mattered to Papa that I was a girl. He taught me to love and understand sports like anyone else, inviting me into a world traditionally set up for men and allowing me to make it my home too. We still talk every weekend, usually catching up on the Oregon Ducks, but more often than not these days our discussions also include the performances of WNBA stars as well.

My relationship with sports wasn't molded in a traditional way. I don't remember our family playing catch together. We didn't go to the park for pickup basketball or spend summers on the tennis courts. Nonetheless, I was drawn to give volleyball and basketball a shot. In truth, I found sports as a refuge—going to practice after school was my way of avoiding loneliness and solitude as a latchkey kid. The adult engagement and interaction with other kids was a means of connection. And as a bonus, I was actually pretty good.

In today's world, where so many parents are involved in their kids' athletic endeavors, making big investments in travel, coaching, and gear, I see access and privilege as a big reason why their children can excel. I was not the kid who was able to join travel teams or afford extra coaching. I struggled with finding transportation and having the needed equipment. Still, I persevered in junior high, making my mark as a good teammate and valuable contributor. But once I no longer lived within walking distance from school, staying for practice required more creativity. I had friends who offered rides when I asked, but it became harder to keep up with the schedule. Even though I was passionate about sports, logistics created barriers for me that I could not solve on my own.

I needed more investment from the adults around me to cultivate my talent in volleyball and basketball. I became interested in other activities that were easier to manage. One of the extracurriculars I gravitated toward was speech and debate. The coach, Daphne Sturtz, saw that I had some natural skill during speech class and encouraged me to join the team. I was enticed by the competitive aspect of it, and Mrs. Sturtz was encouraging, positive, and deeply invested in all of us. She took a girl who was fairly worried about the unpopular decision to join the team and led me all the way to the state championships. To this day, I think my joy of teaching came from learning how to speak in front of others.

I vividly recall one speech that garnered the most awards. It was about the Olympic gymnast Kerri Strug, who performed on the 1996 team known as the "Magnificent Seven." In the final rotation, the United States was on vault and held a lead for the gold over Russia. Kerri was the last to vault for the United States and she fell, badly injuring her ankle. The team was in danger of losing the Olympic title if her second vault didn't go well. Her coach, Bela Karolyi, told her she had to go, despite her obvious injury. She pulled through for the team but collapsed to the ground. Bela carried her to the medal podium before she went to the hospital for a third-degree lateral sprain and tendon damage.

At the time, Kerri's performance was heralded as heroic. She was the epitome of a tough athlete. But in my speech, I argued that it was an injustice that she was compelled to compete despite being so significantly hurt. She didn't have a choice and her coach had made that clear; in his own recounting to the media[5] that day, Bela recalled saying, "'You have to do it, Kerri,'" before going on to explain that "it was a once-in-a-lifetime situation. If it was me, I would go there with a broken leg. I would do anything. This was the gold medal."

My speech called out and questioned what it meant for young girls not to have a voice in their health and their careers. The world-famous coach had all the power, and he was benefiting from the team's success. I knew in my gut that what I was watching on TV was not OK, although I didn't fully understand at that age how many layers of exploitation were at play. I called out the power dynamic and asked fans to reevaluate what we expect from athletes. Little did I know that this speech would foreshadow what awaited me professionally, later in life.

Today, I'm an award-winning senior faculty member at the University of Oregon, in the couples and family therapy graduate program, and a licensed marriage and family therapist, as well as the director of the university's Center for Healthy Relationships at the HEDCO Clinic. As the program's clinical director, I teach and supervise graduate students in their pursuit of becoming mental health therapists. My goal is to teach new clinicians to love this field as much as I do, and I'm conscious of the position of power that I hold as a white ciswoman. How I talk to students, the way I approach course content, and how I give feedback is all done with the understanding that each student has more to them than their academic endeavors. Much like a coach, it's my job to understand the unique needs of each student and adjust. It's never about giving my students shortcuts or not holding them to high standards; it's honoring the fact that we all carry a lot and when we work together, we can all find success.

Clinically, I work with people dealing with self-harm, grief, trauma, and issues of substance use and recovery. I'm also part of the university's athletic mentor program and have served as a mental health consultant for the athletics program and as the chief science officer of the Athletes Mental Health Foundation. In my field, rather than assuming mental health needs mean that something is "wrong" with us, we focus on a systemic understanding. If someone is struggling with depressive symptoms, we explore their relationships and experiences, and often, their circumstances make sense after we understand the larger context. This has led me to think about how, when athletes experience mental health struggles, we can zoom out and see that often they are trying to operate in systems that are exploitative or misogynistic. This perspective adds more to their stories and illustrates why change is not a single person's responsibility, but that of the entire athletic community.

In my career, I've talked with a significant number of athletes, and I've consistently heard about how they don't have the space to discuss their mental health struggles within the systems in which they train and compete. I know that the budgets of most athletic programs don't support hiring enough qualified mental health providers to meet the ever-growing demand (and yes, the mental health providers are often a different budget line from what the football teams are afforded by donors—a frustrating fact about how funds are distributed in athletic departments). Some coaches and staff have said to me in the training sessions I lead that "we don't have any mental health issues; we're all good," a perspective that I know is false. It's like denying you've ever had any player on your team suffer physical injuries: it's impossible. Meanwhile, others acknowledge the problem but just don't know how to help. I have seen firsthand how much athletic programs need from mental health professionals.

It's these moments that have lit my fire. Athletes continue to suffer as some athletic departments do the bare minimum. Women continue to find themselves mistreated and misunderstood. I may have come to this juncture in a different way than Katie, but somehow we've arrived at the same place, and with the same goals and intentions. We want to give women a healthy, supportive place where they are empowered to compete to the best of their abilities, under coaches and systems that foster their success. We can be part of the solution that builds athletes up instead of breaking them down. To do this effectively, athletic systems must acknowledge their power and make space for mental health needs and challenges.

Chapter One

A NEW WAY OF THINKING ABOUT WOMEN'S SPORTS

We can create an environment where female athletes
are set up to succeed from the start.

Teagan is a seven-year-old girl who knows what "being a champion" feels like. She's fallen in love with soccer. There's no mistaking the enthusiasm in her voice when she talks about running around the pitch and scoring goals. By first grade, Teagan already has a dream. "To become an all-star," she says. And if you're wondering what "becoming an all-star" means to the early elementary school crowd, it requires a player to "win lots of games," Teagan explains.

And why shouldn't every seven-year-old girl want that? Girls today have seen the US women's soccer team gain admiration, respect, and popularity not only for winning World Cups and Olympic medals but also for demanding they are paid equitably in return for their skill and talent. They can watch tennis star Coco Gauff break records at the US Open or follow their favorite WNBA teams' regular season games on television—an option that didn't exist a mere fifteen years ago. Even the 2021 Tokyo Olympics were female-focused. From gymnastics to swimming to track and field and more, Team USA had forty-five more women competing at the Summer Games than men and they brought home almost 60 percent of the medals awarded to the American athletes.[1]

In many ways, women's sports have never enjoyed such a devoted following until now, a half century after Title IX became law, providing equal opportunity in federally funded education and sports. And never before have budding female athletes had so many role models and examples of how their athletic feats can be celebrated and recognized. It leaves little wonder why young players like Teagan yearn to become "all-stars" so early.

Even so, it still takes a concerted effort to get these messages and images in front of fans of all ages. Sports remain a vastly male-dominated arena in terms of media coverage, advertising, marketing, and influence. Title IX hasn't changed that, though research released by Wasserman and ESPNW[2] in 2023 shows a bit of progress. In its findings across broadcasts, streaming, social media, and digital publications, women's sports received 15 percent of sports coverage in 2022. Up until recently, most studies showed that men's sports got about 95 percent of total television coverage but didn't account for the many ways and platforms that we watch competition these days. Even so, we still have a long way to go toward equity on the airwaves (however we define them) and on the pay scale, too.

Why does it matter? It reinforces the notion that women aren't as accomplished and their competition is trivial, unworthy of equal attention, and not as entertaining or intense as men's action. That pervasive attitude trickles all the way down to the playground, where we've discovered through our conversations with Teagan and other girls her age that some old-fashioned, boys'-club behavior is still alive and well. Federal policy, as it turns out, doesn't automatically shift cultural norms and attitudes, even after more than fifty years.

Teagan and her friend Everly, who has taken a liking to basketball, report that during recess every day, the boys claim the fields and courts while the girls play tag or use the playground equipment. Even if they wanted to play soccer or shoot some hoops, the girls don't feel welcomed. According to unspoken playground rules, it's not their territory. "That's why the boys are way better," Everly says, "because they get all that extra practice time at recess."

Girls are conditioned early, consciously or not, to understand their place in the athletic world, that their desires and needs are less important. While the opportunities for them to participate have expanded greatly, they are also still playing within systems that were not created by or for female athletes (and likely aren't led by women, either), which can lead to mental health ramifications down the road.

When participation requires the additional burden of advocacy and special permission from a bunch of boys dominating the playing field, it's exhausting and demoralizing. How much would a female athlete's performance improve if she didn't also have to spend her energy fighting for practice time, facilities, and equal status or pay? As more girls devote more of their time to competing, we are increasingly recognizing the short- and long-term repercussions they experience under outdated systems that were never meant to include them.

The message to girls and women on the field of play has always been: Be aggressive, but not too aggressive. Win at all costs, but be polite while you're doing it. Make yourself strong, but not too big. From the beginning, female athletes have performed under these standards and within athletic systems that were created for me. And these systems are still largely led by men. In fact, the percentage of female coaches leading women's teams at the collegiate level has declined from more than 90 percent when Title IX was passed in 1972 to 43 percent fifty years later[3]—a number that has remained mostly stagnant for decades.

The problem? Girls and women at every level encounter unique issues that are largely ignored under the current approaches to training and competition—like puberty, disordered eating, anxiety, depression, and the prevalence of emotional and physical abuse in sports. Now that more female athletes than ever before are participating, we're seeing the consequences in real time. We know that athletes in particular may not look for help out of fear of losing playing time, a scholarship, or their spot on the team. In August 2021, the American College of Sports Medicine reported that only 10 percent of all college athletes with known mental health conditions sought care from a mental health professional.[4] Some don't want to appear less than perfect, weak, or vulnerable. After-all, athletes are trained to persevere, to push through discomfort; they are lauded for their toughness. But we know that when access to mental health resources is available and athletes are encouraged to use them, performance expectations of them can actually increase.

In researching this book, we spoke to hundreds of girls and women, as well as parents, coaches, administrators, officials, sponsors, and fans, to try to pinpoint what is contributing to the obvious decline in mental health among female athletes. Sport is a mirror of society, and the problems seem daunting. The demand for mental-health care providers has outpaced the workforce, and the lack of financial resources further complicates access. According to the 2023 State of Mental Health Report by Mental Health America,[5] one in ten youth in the United States were experiencing depression severely impairing their ability to function at school, home, with family, or in their social lives, and nearly 60 percent of these young people with major depression have not received any treatment because their insurance doesn't cover it or their caregivers can't afford it. When athletes bring untreated mental health issues into a sports environment that exacerbates their symptoms, it's a recipe for the kind of despair and frustration we hear about over and over again.

But we also know that when an athlete finds a sport they love, in a safe and nurturing space, it can provide protection, too. The community, sense of belonging, teamwork, skill-building, and physical activity can ease many symptoms of conditions like depression and anxiety. What girls and women need, however, are sports that are created for them, instead of continuing to survive second-rate versions of the games men play.

Athletes, parents, and coaches can work together to reimagine the female sports experience from the beginning. We can create leagues, shift coaching philosophies, and reform training strategies so that they support the next generation of female all-stars, allowing them to enjoy active lives for far longer, at whatever level their abilities take them.

We know these changes are important because sports can have a profound effect on the trajectory of a girl's life. She can find community, forge a healthy connection with her body, learn how to work with a diverse group of coaches, teammates, and competitors, and better navigate all the pressure and expectations she'll face. It's a place where she'll encounter social and emotional learning, developing empathy for others while establishing and maintaining supportive relationships. And research shows that experience in sports can also translate to professional success later in life: an oft-cited Ernst & Young study found that 94 percent of women who hold C-suite positions in Corporate America played sports and 52 percent of them participated at the collegiate level.[6]

It's clear that sports can lead to a host of positive outcomes. Now we need to examine how we foster and cultivate the experience in equitable ways that don't diminish the joy of participation among girls and women.

It's time to reinvent the female athletic experience, from the youth leagues up through the elite athlete's career. We now know that girls and women do not need to conform to the ways in which male athletes train and compete. We want to create new norms that support the unique mental health needs of female athletes, to create a culture where they can perform and thrive on and off the track, pitch, field, pool, course, mat, rink, or court.

Through the stories of female athletes of all ages and ability levels, the following pages illuminate where it often goes wrong and help girls, women, parents, and coaches understand that they aren't alone in their experiences. We also offer our expertise on how to navigate these issues. And while *The Price She Pays* is more than fifty years overdue, we also expose that we still have a long way to go. We start now.

Chapter Two

DISCOVERING SPORTS

Giving girls a healthy introduction to an active life.

Young girls are the epitome of wonder, energy, and curiosity. In the course of a single Saturday morning, they can go from playing dress-up to tossing a football in the backyard to practicing piano to coloring pictures, and more. For an all-too-brief window of their lives, girls are uninhibited by worries that will eventually creep in, like fear of failure, embarrassment, and comparison traps. They have their own brand of swagger, pushing boundaries and experimenting with all kinds of activities as they are given the chance.

Girls as young as three or four can get a developmental boost from the simplest forms of movement. Unstructured playtime, like tossing a ball in the yard or climbing the jungle gym at the park, allows them to work on their motor skills, coordination, and even mental processing. Learning how to get to the top of the slide and waiting for their turn to go down, for example, also gives them tools to start figuring out social awareness and communication.

According to the American Academy of Pediatrics, toddlers are too young for organized programs,[1] aside from classes they take with their caregivers, but it's not too early to start exposing them to activities like dancing, tumbling, swimming, throwing, catching, or running. Pediatricians recommend that adults join their children at this stage, showing them that moving is fun and feels good. After all, toddlers learn best by copying others.

By the time children reach age six, it's appropriate to find some more organized activities, like t-ball, soccer, martial arts, and gymnastics—programs that teach the fundamentals of the game or activity. This is when they are ready to follow directions, learn new skills, and practice social interactions. The rules should be flexible, though—think smaller fields, smaller equipment, shorter practices and games, and very little focus on scores and competition. Seek out programs that emphasize fun over performance. Children learn soon enough how success is ultimately measured by the masses. Remember Everly, who has already discovered by first grade that she likes winning? She adds that she also enjoys shooting baskets, dribbling, and "zigzagging" on the court. And she lists "snacks" as a reason why she goes to basketball, which is an appropriate response at any age, and an especially poignant one from a seven-year-old.

It's important to allow children to try a variety of activities, if possible, to figure out what captures their passion and attention. Kids shouldn't play anything competitively until they understand that their self-worth is not based on their results. Doing a little research and talking to other parents will uncover the programs that align with that advice. Some children choose to follow in older siblings' footsteps (a carpooling dream, perhaps, but not a reason to push in that direction), while others are influenced by what their parents watch or have played themselves. If a child generally seems happy to go to practice and expresses interest in the sport independent of any adult's prodding, she has found a good fit.

Alice*, for example, was about ten years old when she stood on the side of a local track and watched a group of a dozen other kids take off on a hundred-meter sprint, some of them flaming out halfway through, others pushing full-steam ahead to the finish. The noncompetitive youth program welcomed all abilities from ages ten through thirteen. Her sisters had participated on and off for a couple of years and her parents were avid runners themselves. But Alice wasn't sure if track was for her; she was just there to give it a try. Although she had fun that day, she decided that she liked soccer better. Not only did she enjoy developing ball-handling skills but Alice already had friends on the soccer team, which is often a deciding factor for kids. Her parents' only rule when it came to physical activity was that their children move their bodies for at least thirty minutes a day, whether they chose a brisk walk, family room yoga, games outside, or joined an organized team. No pressure to perform, just a push to form healthy habits early on. How they did it was up to each of them.

Alice's experience was the ideal, though maybe not the norm. At the earliest ages, the reasons why girls like sports are often exactly what they should be: friendships, fun, and movement that makes them feel good. If only we could bottle this moment in time and keep it this pure forever. The introduction to sports is pivotal, and allowing girls to experience healthy environments from the start can set them up for longevity. This sets the stage for how sports will fit into their lives, how they will balance athletics with other priorities like school, friends, and family, and how they'll progress as teammates and athletes in the future. Yet getting into sports is not always as smooth as Alice's experience.

SETTING THE STAGE

When Natalie, who's ten years old, decided to play flag football, the coaches warmly welcomed her to the team. Because she's a girl participating in a traditionally male sport (at least in her area—flag football is growing as an official girls' sport in many school districts across the country), she had to obtain permission from the league to play. Her parents completed additional forms and met with program directors for clearance. We speculate that none of the boys' parents went through the same process, nor would they have to if their sons wanted to try traditionally female sports like synchronized swimming or rhythmic gymnastics. When Natalie attended practice, she felt alone, she says. None of the boys talked to her, and some were just downright rude, making inappropriate comments and gestures because she's their only female teammate. "Boys don't think girls are tough," she observes. "They are always surprised at how I can throw a football."

Natalie, however, remains largely unfazed. Ever since kindergarten, she's demanded her place in boy-dominated spaces. She recalls the time in second grade when she asked an adult recess monitor to help her join a game on the playground after the boys rejected her request. With adult intervention, the group became friendlier and more inclusive. Her takeaway? "I hope boys are taught that girls are equal and can have the same rights." Amen, Natalie.

Experiencing clear gender biases so early in life and finding a way to play sports that feel so exclusive is a heavy lift for such young girls. But for Natalie, it doesn't supersede the joy she feels while playing flag football. Her parents and coaches have her back; they are creating a foundation in which their young athlete feels secure enough in who she is and what she believes to explore the world and make sense of her feelings. She feels supported in her choices. This is part of secure attachment, a concept that we'll visit often in this book, and what allows children to become resilient, insightful, grounded, and connected to themselves—all traits that translate well to athletic pursuits, too, as Natalie matures to higher levels of sport.

During these tween years, girls start to narrow their interests. They may start recognizing their talent in one sport versus another. They may also gravitate to the place where they feel a strong sense of belonging and connection with their friends. Parents, too, will probably begin befriending other team parents, creating an expanded community that involves the entire family.

At this point, sports can also become more competitive and time-consuming—and often require more financial investment. That doesn't mean that these activities have to become any less fun, but the dynamics begin to shift. Weekends are devoted to traveling to competitions, weeknights revolve around practice schedules, and everybody becomes a little more invested in results. Sometimes the general mood in a household is dictated by how the athlete feels about her performance. It's a time when parents want to set their children up for success and maximize their potential, while knowing that pushing too hard can be detrimental. Early specialization can come with consequences like overuse injuries (doing repetitive motions can strain or damage growing muscles, tendons, and bones), mental stress, and burnout. It seems that getting too serious, too early can turn out either really well (Olympic gold! Full-ride scholarship!) or very poorly (hurt, depressed, and spending too much time on the couch) for most kids.

We also know that the cost of participation becomes a big barrier for many kids and their caregivers. According to the 2022 Project Play Report by the Aspen Institute, the average family pays $883 annually for one child's primary sport.[2] Parents in the wealthiest households spend four times more on their child's sport than the lowest-income families. "Bottom line: Children in the U.S. are still having different sports experiences based on money," according to the report.

It never hurts to proceed with caution and allow children to decide how much of themselves they want to give to a specific activity, checking in with them periodically and making sure it's still what they want to do, offering the option to try other sports, too, to avoid those pitfalls like burnout. A 2019 report by the Aspen Institute's Project Play found that the average child spends less than three years playing a sport, quitting by age eleven.[3] The top-cited reasons: the young athlete doesn't think the sport is fun anymore and parents are under pressure to spend thousands of dollars a year, mostly in travel expenses. The research also revealed that kids are typically not quitting one sport to try another—most often, they just lose interest or stop enjoying the experience altogether. The researchers' concerns highlighted that coaches are making excessive demands on young athletes and sports programs aren't accommodating kids who are late bloomers or whose families lack financial resources.

Quinn, for example, tried soccer and gymnastics first around age eleven but decided against both. She didn't like the hours involved in gymnastics, and soccer was a rainy, slippery affair that hurt her shins. She liked volleyball because it was popular, and she discovered she was good at it. But the coaches were discouraging—when she joined, she didn't know the rules yet, so she was separated from her age group. It helped her develop skills, but watching her friends having fun together in a different group was hard. "The coaches would yell at you and make fun of you when you dropped the ball," Quinn says.

She knew that her parents wanted her to keep participating in sports to form healthy habits, but Quinn hasn't always enjoyed the experiences. Her brother had always been involved in sports and she had been under the false impression she might have to do the same to receive the same love and attention. While her parents insisted that she finish the volleyball season she started, they also left the door open for her to try other activities that might be a better fit. Quinn came to realize that she could choose her own adventure, independent of her brother's path. She's also come to understand that it doesn't have to feel like a pressure-filled endeavor, she says, so she's settled on track, where she's not required to compete if she doesn't want to. "The coach is the PE teacher and he's a loud, big, bossy man," she says. "But it feels fair and it pushes my limits. The coaches don't make us do anything we don't want to do." Another important factor for Quinn and her friends: unlike the volleyball coach, the track coaches allowed bathroom breaks when athletes decided they needed them (the volleyball coaches, on the other hand, didn't allow them to visit the bathroom without explicit permission), which are critical for girls her age who are just starting to get their periods.

Later, we'll talk about how puberty also influences the female athletic progression (or too often puts a sudden stop to that progression). But for now, in these early years, we know that girls are absorbing a lot. They're learning the norms of training and competition, observing and experiencing how athletes are treated, understanding what coaches expect of the team and the individuals on it, and regulating their emotions through it all. Often, they're looking at older girls within the league or club and starting to comprehend what's coming next and how the star athletes emerge (or forming their own perceptions about how they gain playing time or achieve other measures of success, depending on the sport). Everly has already noticed, for example, that the kids whose parents are coaches receive more attention than other players, but she's still motivated to work hard because she believes her improving skills will eventually garner recognition, too.

Even at this early stage of sports, we start treating young people like athletes. We focus on practice and game schedules, how they perform, if they're physically healthy, and team dynamics. Their identity gets tied to their athletic endeavors quickly: "She's a gymnast" or "she's a swimmer" or "she's a soccer player," for example. Although it's good to appreciate and encourage their participation, we also want to make sure girls know that they're valued as whole humans, too. When the inevitable ups and downs of sport happen—injuries, for example—and temporarily take an athlete out of their element and routine, we still want them to know their worth as people outside of sport. Instead of asking, "How was practice?" ask, "How are you?" first. This can prompt her to think not just about her physical condition but also shed insight into her mental health, too. So often, athletes are taught to dissociate—to follow directions, focus, compartmentalize, and use the "mind over matter" philosophy to push through discomfort. All of that can lead to athletic greatness and celebrated performances, but it also teaches athletes to disconnect from themselves and their emotions, which can become detrimental to psychological well-being in the long term.

The Women's Sports Foundation notes that by age fourteen, girls drop out of sports at twice the rate of boys.[4] The reasons, the foundation says, are varied. Many girls lack access to transportation and can't walk safely to practices and games. Others sense a social stigma—girls are often still bullied or antagonized for being athletic and discriminated against based on real or perceived sexual orientation and gender identity. And, of course, as girls grow up and no longer play on mixed-gender teams, they notice that the quality of the experience declines—the equipment is subpar, practices are held at inconvenient times to gain access to facilities, coaches are disinterested in leading female teams, or their coaching styles don't match how girls develop and learn.

Jamar, whose sixteen-year-old daughter plays lacrosse and soccer, believes her participation should "bring more joy than agony." He loves watching and cheering her on, and although his friends give their kids incentives (like cash) to improve their stats, he avoids putting such a big focus on those achievements. "I want my kids to play because they love it, not because they earn money or attention," he says.

We applaud Jamar's approach. The first ten years of athletic life should remain as pure and joyful as possible. Learning tools and skills at this point will serve them the rest of their lives; girls can harness a lot of confidence through sports if they are allowed to let their passion drive their participation.

TRANSGENDER YOUTH IN SPORTS

Starting in 2020, states across the country began passing legislation barring transgender girls from participating in girls' sports, as well as banning gender-affirming health care for trans youth. Those who support these laws say that they're trying to "protect women's sports," but at the same time, these advocates haven't paid much attention to fixing issues like equal pay, equal access, more balanced media coverage, or sexual harassment and abuse of female athletes, for example.

As groups like Athlete Ally point out, these laws create unsafe environments for all kids. Many states will have to determine eligibility for girls' sports by testing chromosomes, hormone levels, or inspecting anatomy. We'll begin to see these kinds of invasions of privacy whenever an athlete—transgender or not—appears "too masculine." Inevitably it will further diminish girls' participation if the threat of physical examination is added to the mix of barriers girls already face.

Although many of the people advocating for bans on transgender kids' participation claim their presence is unfair, they fail to recognize other inequities, like kids who grow faster or families who can pay for private coaching, for example. In the meantime, we know that very few young athletes fall into this demographic. In the United States, 1.4 percent of youths ages thirteen to seventeen identify as transgender, according to a study from UCLA's Williams Institute,[5] not all of them are female, and not all of them play sports, disproving the narrative that boys are flocking to female sports to win our trophies.

The medical providers we spoke with agreed that participating in organized sports is not typically a priority for youths who are exploring transitioning. They are navigating complex, life-changing decisions that tend to eclipse the importance of athletics. Andrés Larios Brown, licensed marriage and family therapist at Encircle, which offers mental health support to LGBTQ+ youths and their families, says that LGBTQIA+ people often fear sports, which have historically been places of hurt and exclusion. It can feel daunting to navigate deeply gendered spaces, like locker rooms, and teams based on sex assigned at birth. All of it can prevent transgender and nonbinary youths from even exploring the possibility.

But we do know that inclusion is the humanitarian choice. The Trevor Project, a suicide prevention organization for lesbian, gay, bisexual, transgender, queer, and questioning young people, published a peer-reviewed, qualitative study that looked at sports participation among 294 transgender high school girls. The research showed that 68 percent have chosen not to play sports,[6] mostly because of fears of bullying and harassment from peers and coaches (and, anecdotally from news reports, we're guessing parents, too), which means they miss out on the benefits like increased self-esteem, fun, friends, better grades, and higher educational opportunities.

"Policies that seek to ban transgender youth from sports only serve to heighten experiences of stigma and reduce the ability of youth to receive the positive physical, social, and emotional benefits of sports," the Trevor Project reports.

WHY THE CULTURE OF SPORTS MATTERS

Every sport has its own culture and when children are exploring which ones they want to pursue, families need to decide if the environment aligns with their lifestyles and values. Some sports require multiple practices a day, while others rely on before-school sessions (sometimes as early as 5:00 a.m.) because that's when facilities like pools or ice rinks are available. Some are travel- and tournament-heavy, requiring families to devote entire weekends (and considerable budgets) to the pursuit.

Aside from the time and financial commitments, though, parents should pay close attention to other, often more subtle norms that are fostered within a club, league, or the sport in general. How do coaches talk about success? Is it win-at-all costs or is it measured in other ways, too, like improvement, teamwork, leadership, and attendance? What about nutrition and recovery? Do athletes understand why fueling is important and why their bodies also need rest? Do they feel like they can speak up if they need a break or might have an injury? What kind of relationships do coaches have with their athletes? Is it marred by favoritism or is it marked by positive communication, mutual respect, and trust?

In recent years we've learned more than ever about how sport cultures have been harmful, especially for women and girls. The US gymnastics case that revealed that athletes were sexually abused by Dr. Larry Nassar, is, of course, one of the most notable. The investigation also uncovered that coaches and officials did nothing to protect athletes, despite knowing that abuse was taking place, and revealed a host of other systemic problems—coaching practices that included berating athletes for gaining weight and pushing athletes to train and compete on broken bones, for instance. In 2022, former US attorney general Sally Yates investigated[7] allegations of other forms of abusive behavior and sexual misconduct in women's professional soccer and discovered an array of problems that didn't begin or end at the very top of the sport, either. "Abuse in the National Women's Soccer League is rooted in a deeper culture in women's soccer, beginning in youth leagues, that normalizes verbally abusive coaching and blurs the boundaries between coaches and players," according to the report.

It shouldn't take a hundred gymnasts coming forward or an investigation by the nation's top law enforcement officer to figure out whether your child is committing to a sport that provides a safe, healthy, and happy environment. But, at the youth level, it takes parental involvement.

Caroline* became a devoted hockey player at a young age, which wasn't a surprise because her father was a pro player. But her path to the collegiate level was challenging, to say the least. For years, she woke before dawn to go to physically demanding practices where the coach yelled obscenities at the players, often criticized their bodies, and when they lost games, he punished them, demanding that they remain on the ice, sprinting back and forth until many of them vomited. Caroline, who is Asian American, encountered racist abuse from competitors during games and on social media, but her coach did nothing to protect her.

Caroline's mother, who had experience as an athletic administrator, tried to talk with the coach and point out the concerns about her daughter's experience and his behavior. She didn't get much support from other parents, who feared that if they intervened, their children would lose playing time or suffer other repercussions. The coach was admired and celebrated within the community because of his winning record. Nobody wanted to cross him. But Caroline's mom believed that no matter how elite the league was, it wasn't worth her daughter's well-being. She pulled Caroline from the program, showing her that no athletic goals or dreams were worth enduring abuse, mistreatment, and bullying. Caroline, who went on to compete in college, accepted her mother's decision at the time.

In any sport, girls will encounter the power imbalance between coach and athlete. In Caroline's case, she had the added challenge of being a young, female athlete of color, coached by an older white man who she felt was sexist and racist. She needed an advocate, and thankfully her parents were able to teach her that her core values and identity were far more important than athletic glory. It was an unsafe environment in which athletes, including Caroline, were afraid of the coach. That kind of fear-based leadership doesn't foster respect or trust, and it's harmful to the athletes' mental health, exacerbating anxiety, depression, and possibly other symptoms like self-harm and suicidal ideation.

In the best-case scenarios, girls will find teams that develop not just their physical fitness but also allow them to enjoy the process, cultivate their self-esteem, and learn that the pay-off for hard work isn't always tied to winning or perfect performances—that losing isn't the same as failing. Before she gets too deep into her sport, she deserves to experience a healthy relationship with her coaches and find team values that reflect her own. She should know what a safe sport looks and feels like, and she should feel empowered to seek out an advocate if necessary.

Parents and caregivers play the most important role in shaping these experiences by observing how the team communicates and interacts at games, watching how players are treated by their peers and coaches, noticing what behaviors are accepted and modeled, and talking with athletes about what they're experiencing and how they feel about it. Other questions to ask your athlete consistently include: What did you enjoy about practice today? What's something your coach said that you liked? Is there anything that your coach said or did today that you didn't like? Not only will the answers help you learn about the culture of the team, but they'll also provide an opportunity to offer support and feedback. It also allows your girl to know that you're there to help her through disappointments and will also celebrate moments of improvements and achievements. These lines of communication become the norm as she grows and develops throughout her athletic career.

The Yates report on soccer underscores the need to pay attention early and create expectations for what a healthy environment looks like from the start: "The ubiquity of certain kinds of sexist or demeaning remarks as 'tough coaching' normalized verbal and emotional abuse. Overwhelming numbers of players, coaches, and [United States Soccer

Federation] staff observed that women players are conditioned to accept and respond to abusive coaching behaviors as youth players. By the time they reach the professional level, many do not recognize the conduct as abusive."

Soccer and gymnastics are not the only sports to uncover mistreatment of athletes, of course. But they illustrate how win-at-all-costs sport systems can become toxic, beginning at the youth level and continuing on through the professional ranks. From the playground to the travel team, parents and caregivers should understand where it can go wrong for girls like Teagan, Everly, Natalie, and Caroline, and be prepared to do something about it.

Chapter Three

PARENTING AN ATHLETE

The role of caregivers is pivotal and sometimes precarious as children become more serious about their athletic endeavors.

You've seen those commercials during the Olympics and Paralympics. The tearjerkers paying homage to all the mothers who have reared the best athletes in the world. The moms who tenderly roused their children from bed, flipping pancakes and shepherding them to predawn practices. The ones who cajoled their offspring to keep trying, picking them up after tough losses, appearing as the stalwart supporter through thick and thin. The mothers who nursed their growing prodigies back to health and happiness through the decades of setbacks, injuries, and illnesses.

Then, cue the shot of the proud parent, now a little grayer, cheering the long-awaited victory from the middle of the stands, donning the unmistakable red, white, and blue apparel. The ending is always the same. A medal, a teary embrace, and a simple, sentimental message: "Thank you, Mom."

It's the entire fairy tale (minus due credit to other caregivers, including fathers) in two emotionally intense minutes, selling the Olympic dream (and a few personal hygiene products to boot). Procter &

Gamble knows its audience and how to tug at the heartstrings of every family who's raising an aspiring Olympian or Paralympian. And even if the hopes don't run quite so high in your living room, chances are that most people can relate to the underlying message of the campaign: caregivers are the stewards of their athlete's greatest ambitions—or, at least, they strive to be.

What those 120 seconds don't show is just *how* those parents did it all so perfectly. That's because they didn't, of course; nobody has a secret formula for raising a gold medalist or even a local soccer league's star goalkeeper. Neither do these ads show the late-night squabbles over unwashed uniforms, missing cleats, or unfinished homework. In real life, the happy ending, however it's defined, comes with many challenges along the way: How do you help your athlete build a foundation of self-esteem that will sustain her through those disappointments, pressures, injuries, and more? When do you step back? When do you step in? How do you support her without pushing too much (or too little)? The role of the athlete's parent is, at times, fraught. And not all athletes have somebody who takes that kind of interest in their passion, either.

Caroline, the young hockey player we met in chapter 2, who experienced mistreatment and racism on the ice before changing leagues, was fortunate to come from a home that nurtured her love of sports from the beginning. Sam*, her mother, wanted Caroline to advance to the highest levels if she chose to, but not by sacrificing her emotional and physical well-being. Sam knew that allowing Caroline to play for the more elite, but abusive, team would ultimately teach her to accept that kind of treatment later in life, whether in sports, relationships, or the workforce. It was about more than hockey. To Sam, it was instilling core values in her children through sports and other experiences, emphasizing the development of the whole person over the development of the athlete.

Such a decision to steer clear of a toxic sports environment may seem obvious from the outside, but it's not always the clearest choice when you're in it (after all, Sam didn't find a lot of public support among the team's parents when she voiced the concerns that she knew they shared). It is through sports that we teach kids to keep pushing. And we invest a lot in what we think will help children get to the next level. The intentions are almost always good, but in today's youth sports culture, it's also easy for adults to get wrapped up in the possibilities, from making prestigious travel teams, securing starting positions, and earning college scholarships to, yes, maybe even tasting professional or Olympic glory one day.

Parents want the best for their children, but they sometimes need a reality check.

The truth is, most athletic careers don't progress beyond the high school level; according to NCAA statistics, of the 394,105 high school girls playing soccer in 2020, for example, only 2.4 percent moved on to compete for a Division I college team,[1] and only 1.3 percent of female high school basketball players advanced to an NCAA DI opportunity that same year. Fewer than 2 percent of all high school athletes are offered athletic scholarships each year, according to NCAA statistics. In other words, from the start, participating in sports has to be about more than earning a spot on an elite college team, and it's a caregiver's job to keep that perspective.

One pro endurance athlete we spoke with remembers how her competitive fires were stoked by her father from a young age. Like many girls, she started out playing soccer but ended up discovering her love of running on the field. She made the transition to track and field and cross-country naturally in middle school, but it wasn't always easy to feel like she was living up to expectations. "When I started showing promise and interest with running, he was all in with me and he'd take me out to do workouts and runs and got really invested," the athlete told us. "He has been a really big part of my athletic journey, but also I have felt pressure from him during various periods."

As she advanced through high school and eventually competed for a Division I program, her parents remained supportive, though her father took disappointing performances personally at times. "I know that my dad loves me unconditionally, but I think sometimes it has felt conditional related to my achievement, whereas with my mom, that's *really* unconditional, you know? She is always the first person to say, 'You know, you don't have to do this anymore.' He's never forced me to keep going, but I've gotten so much of my affirmation from him related to achievement."

It's normal for parents to feel excitement and investment in their children's activities, but when taken to an excessive degree, that investment can make it difficult for kids to define themselves outside of their sports, especially when they feel their own caregiver's identity is also wrapped up in their performance. It's important for young athletes to see that adults have other parts of themselves that are important, so that they, too, can cultivate many facets of their lives.

DISCOVERING YOUR FAMILY'S SPORTS VALUES

Core values are a fundamental part of who you are and should easily translate to sports. Those athletes who are able to nail down those values on the field of play and in the stands as fans will find themselves grounded, connected, and true to themselves in the heat of competition and away from it.

In therapy, one of our favorite tools is a values exercise. It taps into your beliefs and can be used anytime you want.

1. Make a list of ten values that resonate with you. If you're stuck, brainstorm examples of values like integrity, compassion, and connection, for example, and choose the ones that ring true. Then pick a verb that makes values actionable, such as "promote flexibility" or "act with integrity."

2. Define each value and what it means to you. The definition gives the value more meaning and connection.

3. Over the course of a few weeks or a month, try to eliminate some of the values—the ones that don't seem to align with your daily life.

4. Narrow the list to three to five core values and notice how you feel when you embody them.

5. Practice one phrase each day in your daily routine or spend a month trying out a few different ones together. The goal is to keep the values that feel good and integrate them into the way you operate within the family's sport life and outside of it.

CREATING SECURITY

We've already mentioned the concept of attachment, and it's an essential component of raising a healthy female athlete. We'll focus on three kinds of attachment between caregiver and child: secure, avoidant, and anxious. We're aiming for the secure variety, which means a caregiver is creating opportunities for a child to learn about themselves and what they need, while providing guidance, approval, validation, and comfort. In a secure attachment, a young person knows that everything will be OK, even when a situation does not feel OK, because they've been shown consistently that they're worthy of love and care (usually since infancy—when they cried, their caregiver tended to their needs, figuring out if they were hungry, needed a diaper change, or were sick, for example).

Cultivating such a relationship with a budding female athlete is a collaborative and evolving process. What a five-year-old requires from a parent is much different than a teenager, but all children need a consistent sense of safety and security from the primary adult(s) in their lives, regardless of the circumstances or the emotions involved. In turn, they're likely to develop higher self-esteem and confidence throughout their lives.

Speaking of emotions, a telltale sign of secure attachment is the ability to acknowledge and process difficult emotions, instead of stuffing them down, ignoring them, internalizing, or reacting negatively to them. Playing sports induces all kinds of emotions, the ups and downs, joys, defeats, embarrassments, mistakes. Children can't play any sport and not feel them, but what matters is what they do with them. A caregiver is the first to set an example; it's called coregulation. Parents can calm their children through their own tone of voice, body movements, facial expressions, and reactions. What does your athlete see or hear from you after she misses an important free throw or falls off the balance beam? Is it reassurance? Is it panic? Anger? If parents know how to regulate their emotions, they can coregulate with their children, who trust them to be predictable and consistent (hopefully in a productive, supportive way).

To be clear, coping with emotions does not make anybody "soft," which is a concern we've heard from a startling number of coaches, any time the subject of mental health arises. Helping young athletes learn to shift gears, trust others, and feel supported furthers their love of sport and helps them grow into complete humans and better athletes. Part of regulation is knowing how to cope with the feeling of discomfort, a sensation that athletes will feel constantly as they push their perceived physical and mental boundaries. Athletes don't have to be "hard" people—but that doesn't mean they are "soft," either. When kids receive no validation of their feelings, the result is avoidant attachment. If they say, "My coach was really mean to me today," and their caregiver retorts, "Get used to it. Your boss will be mean to you one day, too," they end up distancing themselves from others and are unlikely to seek support when they need it. And when a child learns to suppress what they're feeling, they'll never learn how to work through sadness, anger, or disappointment.

Kathy's daughter, Kate, was a decorated competitive cheerleader and competed in collegiate acrobatics and tumbling, where she won championship titles. They have always shared a close relationship—Kathy was a reliable presence throughout Kate's athletic career. But one of the most important ways she supported Kate was by giving her space after practices and meets, especially after those that didn't go well. Even when Kathy wanted to talk or check in, she knew that Kate preferred to decompress and process her experiences on her own before she discussed them with her mom. "It felt respectful and caring," Kate says. "I wasn't pressured to talk about how it went, knowing that my mom would be there, regardless, when I was ready."

When it felt right, Kathy often asked Kate open-ended questions, like how she felt at practice or how she thought the competition went—that way, Kate could drive the conversation in whatever way she wanted. If Kathy knew that the team or Kate as an individual athlete had been working on specific aspects of their performance, she'd ask how it was going. If Kathy had attended the event, she'd point out a few positive observations, even something like, "the team seemed really supportive of each other today."

"Regardless of performance, I'd always tell Kate that I was proud of her and love to see her out there doing what she loves to do," Kathy says.

A child with secure attachment knows that love and support aren't contingent on outcomes like wins or losses because their parents are there no matter what. That doesn't mean that parents should ignore less desirable or bad outcomes, but they can create a household environment that doesn't always rise and fall based on wins, losses, injuries, and triumphs. Disappointments are inevitable, and athletes like Kate will get through them with more ease because her mother will understand them and support her either way. "As a parent, I had to allow Kate to have those frustrations and disappointments and work through them," Kathy says. "And at times I'd offer guidance, but most of the time I knew she needed to work through them on her own."

WHAT IS ATTACHMENT?

Simply put, attachment is the bond that forms between children and their caregivers. It's important because it helps us learn how to form close relationships in adulthood. Children look to the adults in their lives for guidance, approval, validation, and comfort, especially when they feel stressed or threatened in some way. Those who have formed a secure foundation give their children the confidence to explore the world around them.

Early attachment research measured whether a child feels that their caregiver would be there to take care of them when needed. Attachment develops when the parent or guardian gives consistent warm, sensitive feedback to their child and provides a sense of safety and comfort.

Secure attachments allow children to learn about themselves and their own needs. As adults, we can help them with this process by asking them what they think, how they feel, and giving them an opportunity to share.

MANAGING THE PRESSURES

An entire Oscar-winning movie was released in 2022 about one of the most celebrated parent-athlete relationships: Richard Williams and his tennis star daughters, Venus and Serena. While most parents aren't going to coach their daughters to become two of the most famous athletes on the planet, the movie *King Richard* reveals a few ideas about how to support kids who show talent early on. Richard Williams famously pulled his daughters from the junior tennis circuit in an effort to preserve their mental and physical well-being for the long haul. "Everyone's like, 'Well how do you play tennis for so long?' It's because we weren't raised in an environment where it was something that we abhorred," Serena said in an interview with *Harper's Bazaar*.[2]

That statistic from the Aspen Institute's Project Play report we cited earlier sticks with us, so we'll repeat it: the average child spends less than three years playing a sport, quitting by age eleven because it's not fun anymore. A host of variables can make sports less fun for kids, and unfortunately, parents are one factor. As children grow and improve in their sport, they can begin to feel that their worth is tied to their performance. That's a form of anxious attachment and it leads young athletes to feel nervous and hesitant, wondering how they might make their parents or caregivers happy that day. It generates low self-esteem and lack of confidence because the love and support that a child feels depends on their performance on the field of play. They sense that a parent is happy when they win and disappointed in a loss.

Ryan* admits he was one of "those parents." His two daughters are now adults, but back when they played volleyball, the family maximized every opportunity to push them toward athletic success. At first, they dabbled in gymnastics, diving, swimming, and soccer, but in high school they decided to specialize in volleyball. Between school teams and club teams, it quickly became an all-consuming, year-round endeavor. They frequently traveled from their home base in California to Colorado and Nevada on the weekends, arriving home late on Sunday nights just in time to launch into a new week and do it all over again. The family remembers it as "seven years of chaos." They had no breathing room between volleyball, schoolwork, social events, and Ryan's growing business. The days were long and full.

With such a big commitment to the sport, Ryan expected excellence from his daughters, as well as their teammates, coaches, and other parents. He frequently felt frustrated and consumed by outcomes; at games, he often yelled at the girls to try harder and do better. The gym was always full of such intensity. Parents and spectators yelled at the refs, and the temperature was hot. At one tournament, when the team fell short, the female coach piled the entire team in a bathroom stall and yelled, "This is where you belong if you're going to play like shit." The coach had no boundaries and criticized the athletes constantly. In one instance, Ryan observed his daughter on the receiving end of the coach's ire, which finally led Ryan to step in and tell the coach to never treat her like that again. Though Ryan could get overzealous and lose his cool at times, he also couldn't stand by and say nothing when another adult crossed the line. His own behavior, in addition to the coach's tactics, illustrate so much of the current culture in youth sports. Everything seems intense, and the adults in the room don't always engage in appropriate ways.

Ryan says his goal "was to ensure his girls grew up to be strong, successful women." Now adults, Ryan's daughters are mothers and business owners. His oldest says that sports made her stronger. "I learned how to work through hard things and the true meaning of teamwork, confidence, grit, and perseverance," she says. "It taught me how to push limits, become depleted, and show up anyway to follow through on my commitments."

Today, Ryan reflects on how tough he was and how that chapter of his family's life was extreme. "All I know is that I love my daughters and who they have become," he says. "They are intense, and I wish they were softer at times, but that would make them perfect and that isn't possible. It's nice to look back and know we would do most of it all over again."

Setting expectations for athletic children can be complicated, as Ryan and his family learned; their experience came with positives and negatives, like most people's involvement in sports. A lot of parents share Ryan's goal of teaching kids how to be strong and get through the obstacles and challenges they'll face "in the real world." This can also lead to an avoidant attachment for young athletes, who can become extremely independent, overly self-reliant, and uncomfortable with intimate connections. These are the people with an intense "mind of over matter" mentality: their caregivers are not there to talk through their needs or emotions, so these athletes often don't seek support from others because they've been taught to tough it out and push through challenges on their own.

Often, we hear that parents have "sacrificed a substantial amount of time and money" into sports for their kids. With those investments, they have high expectations. Instead of experiencing the joy of seeing their child engage in teamwork, physical fitness, and play, it becomes a transactional experience. They want to see performance, ample playing time, and advancement. The fun of sports drains quickly and is replaced with pressure and discord—and sometimes resentment, too. These kinds of expectations become more about the adult's return-on-investment instead of allowing kids to flourish on their own terms.

Kailani* is a collegiate track and field athlete in the south who grew up with her sisters, as well as many cousins who are close in age. She didn't see her father a lot as a child but had good relationships with her mom and grandparents. She and her extended family all played sports and it was a central aspect of family life. Before taking to running, Kailani danced, participated in theater, and watched her siblings play basketball. Her mom wanted to give her kids the opportunity to participate in sports and other extracurricular activities in a meaningful way—something she didn't have as a child. "My mom made us go to our siblings' games because you never knew what could happen. It could be their best game ever and having your family in the stands makes a big difference."

Looking back, Kailani is glad she came from a family that was supportive of each other's participation in sports, but she also struggled with feelings of inadequacy when she believed that one of her relatives was a better athlete than she was. She often cried. Coming from a large extended family who were all talented, it was difficult to field the comments from family and friends, and internally, Kailani fell into her own comparison traps. Although caregivers like Kailani's mom and extended family have good intentions, they sometimes forget that children are wired to want to please them, even as they grow older and leave for college. For Kailani, this meant that she always felt pressure to perform when she was standing on the start line. And while pressure in sport is not a bad thing (nor can any athlete avoid it), the source of her anxiety was not wanting to disappoint anybody. "The family pressure and their reactions can take you down," she says. Instead of focusing on her races, Kailani has often felt nervous and scared. Her coping mechanism has been, in great part, prayer; her family "doesn't do mental health."

One of the greatest tools that adults can use in supporting their athletes is *curiosity*. Ask about their experiences without trying to change the circumstances or solve problems for them. How does that athlete think their experience could improve? Curiosity helps children learn to trust their instincts and share more of what they're going through. It also lets them know that they're never enduring their circumstances alone. So when assessing a program, performance, coach, or league, start by asking questions that give athletes the opportunity to express how they feel about their experiences.

In Kailani's case, the transition to college and competing at a higher level was difficult, and now away from family and in a new environment, she sought out mental health support. When she explained to her parents what she was going through, she was initially met with resistance. They didn't understand that healing from her depression wasn't a matter of just overcoming sadness and getting back to academics and training. It was hard for her to explain something in which they didn't seem to have any interest. Kailani began taking antidepressants and slowly helped her family learn more about her condition, she says. "When you can talk about it more, you can normalize it," Kailani says. "Not everyone will completely get it or understand, but they can definitely try and learn." In fact, Kailani's dad has now also sought out therapy himself, inspired by his daughter's experience. By sharing what she was going through, she made mental health accessible to him. "One conversation can shape possibility," Kailani says.

Parents can always play a big part in supporting the mental health of their children, of course, but it's much easier while they're living at home, where a parent or caregiver can directly observe their fluctuations in mood and behavior. A parent notices when communication patterns change, or an athlete seems irritable or preoccupied, or whether a child means it when she says she's "fine" (the stock response we expect). Mental health is still stigmatized, and kids realize that. But we can explain to them from an early age that if they're feeling depressed, it's a condition that is just as treatable—and as important to their success—as a knee injury, for example. If they get the help they need, they'll recover and return to competition feeling better and ready to perform. Again, if emotions are an acceptable topic of family conversation, children will accept challenges as normal and share that they're stressed or sad.

Families can't prevent mental health conditions—and when athletes move out, they start to rely more on teammates, coaches, and trainers as their daily points of contact. However, no matter what age, when a child watches a caregiver work through their own emotions and challenges, whether it's seeking therapy or coping with a work crisis or an irritating customer service phone call, they're given an example of how to do so themselves (or in Kailani's case, she saw that her actions could set a positive example for her father, too). It translates to the field of play.

NAVIGATING PARENTAL INVOLVEMENT

Games, races, and competition happen fast, and mistakes are made. Refs make controversial calls. A lot of emotion is cycling through an athlete at all times. Can they stay focused and continue to work hard as all of this occurs? For athletes to resist reactive tendencies they have to learn how to regulate their emotions at early stages in their development. It's best if they learn this away from sports, but it is certainly a skill that will translate to the field of play and serve them well. We don't want to condition young athletes to not feel any emotions, but we do want them to learn how to cope with those feelings as they identify them. When we resist our feelings, they exacerbate. It's like when we throw too many ingredients into a pot of soup—it overflows. When we feel emotions, giving them time to simmer, they become less powerful, we become more responsive, and we are less reactive; we make room for other feelings.

Katie's oldest child, Camden, for example, found himself in a situation that made him angry, triggered by a medical appointment. Though at seven years old it would be normal and expected for him to lose his temper and react with perhaps tears or anger, instead he paused and took a few deep breaths. He had learned from Mrs. R., his teacher, that deep breaths are "healthiest for me, and my thoughts are just trying to trick me out of doing the hard thing." That's advanced thinking for a young child and a strategy that most adults would do well to learn, too. Katie imagines that Camden will utilize the technique throughout his life and, of course, in his athletic endeavors. Whether it's the excitement of a hockey game, perfecting his backflip, or learning how to wakeboard, Katie has already witnessed this in action. Camden is adept at regulating his thoughts and actions as the emotions swirl around him: as he makes his own mistakes or experiences a win, he relies on the tools he's learned from the adults in his life, like Mrs. R., to build resiliency and confidence.

To their credit, Mrs. R and her husband, Mark, have a lot of experience in helping children like Camden and other young athletes regulate emotions. Their two daughters, ages eleven and thirteen, are active middle schoolers and have played a variety of sports as they've grown up. Mrs. R. was an avid soccer player through college and her girls have followed in her footsteps. She coached their teams from kindergarten through fifth grade with the philosophy that sports should be fun for everybody, and kids that age should be allowed to explore their options to follow their hearts in whatever direction they feel pulled. Soccer and other sports for Mrs. R.'s daughters have been optional—something they should want to do, not be expected to do. The emphasis remains on commitment, not competition. Show up for the entire season, connect with the team, but don't worry about the outcome of the games.

As their daughters have grown up and continued to enjoy soccer, Mark has found his spot. He brings the dog to the games, and they spectate from the end of the field, away from the crowd of parents, which he finds is a more enjoyable way to watch all the kids compete. It's intentional—Mark knows the intensity that escalates on the sidelines, and he doesn't like to yell much. In fact, his daughters have requested that their parents don't holler when they play. Mrs. R. and Mark have respected the boundaries their daughters have set. In their household, it's about the process of practicing soccer and the values that they're developing through sports. The adults have let go of any instinct to micromanage that process for their children and realize that their kids are also individuals—their experiences, skills, and growth in sports will differ.

The athletes we've spoken to mostly wish their parents would just watch and keep the yelling to a minimum. They usually don't hear it anyway or, if they do, they find it mortifying. Some even intentionally block their parents' voices out when they're competing. Do we really want our kids learning how to ignore us in an effort to play more effectively? The perspective from adults matters and caregivers set the tone regarding how sports are integrated into family life. To what extent are parents involved and how does the family want to experience this aspect of life together? Looking down the road, how do parents want their children to reflect on their youth sport experiences?

Meredith, a mother of two teen girls and a licensed clinical social worker, was encouraged to participate in sports as a child, and in turn, she's cultivating the same experience for her daughters, who have vastly different preferences when it comes to physical activity. Her older daughter isn't interested in competition of any kind, though after trying a variety of activities to boost confidence, she found she enjoys running—the movement feels good and it reduces her stress. She sets her alarm for 5:15 a.m., sometimes planning routes with friends or holiday jogs to look at the lights in the neighborhoods. On the other hand, Meredith's younger daughter thrives on intensity and competition. She loves to sharpen her skills and move to the next level, relishing the opportunity to play any sport.

Meredith's younger daughter has decided that she likes soccer best, but it's been a challenging transition as she's gotten older. Not long ago, Meredith dropped her daughter off for a tryout to make a new team, in a league that was more competitive. When Meredith returned, she knew something was different. Her typically peppy, confident girl appeared depleted and somber. Meredith scanned the sidelines, where she sensed tension from the parents who stayed to watch. They were pensive, taking notes, and the coaches were yelling criticism toward the field.

As her daughter and her friend got in the car, they were sure they wouldn't make the team. They were sullen and disappointed. And Meredith found herself also feeling defeated. She and other mothers shared their stress-related responses to the situation. Some even broke out in rashes—over a youth soccer team. It then occurred to Meredith that if she felt this way, how must her daughter feel? How was she coping? Her daughter ended up making the team but ultimately decided to transfer to a different league. She wanted a place where the focus was on teamwork, skill development, and positive reinforcement.

Meredith's daughter is now thriving in an environment that is still intense but where athletes are treated with more dignity and respect: coaches give direction instead of criticism, for example. The parents aren't taking notes on the sidelines but are supportive of the entire group and what they can achieve together. Meredith decided the goal for her family was to cultivate a life of movement, through programs and teams led with the kind of integrity and values they believed in.

FROM PARENT TO COACH (AND BACK AGAIN)

Parents who volunteer their time as youth sports coaches are the lifeblood of the whole operation. So many leagues and community teams would not exist without them. But we know that the role of parent and the role of coach are different, and sometimes it's difficult to reconcile the two, not only for our own children but for the other kids on the team, too. Here are some factors to keep in mind if you decide to lead your daughter's team:

- First, ask your child if she has reservations about you taking on the role of coach. Know that your kids never want to let you down or reject you, so you'll have to encourage them to be honest and express how they really feel about the idea. Keep the conversation open and check in about it more than once.

- Set clear expectations from the beginning, before the season starts, letting your child know that you will treat everybody on the team fairly and equally. You should explain at practice or during a game that you won't be able to drop everything to attend to your child's immediate needs and that because you're leading the group doesn't mean she'll get more playing time, unless she earns it like any other team member. Bring it up at the first practice with the group: let the team know that your daughter is a player and reassure them that you'll treat everybody the same. Leave the door open to feedback, too—to avoid any hint of favoritism, maybe you're actually being harder on your child than you might be on the other kids. Allow your child an opportunity to share that observation. If you have an assistant coach, let that person take more of the lead on communicating with your child.

- Discuss how your role will change from coach to parent after games and practices are over. When you're driving home together, you'll naturally talk about how things went, but don't go overboard (your child isn't your assistant coach, after all). Listen to your daughter as a parent instead of a coach, ask questions about how she feels about how it went, and don't be too eager to share your own perceptions with her. If she had a bad game, reassure her that your love and support are steadfast and never dependent on performance. At home, talk about other topics and let conversations about sports take a back seat.

- Know when to retire. Your daughter will grow and progress with exposure to other coaches who have other philosophies and expertise, so after a season or two, resume your position in the stands and just be her parent. Let her know that you have loved the bonding and time spent together, but you are looking forward to supporting her in a different way.

KEEPING DOORS OPEN

When parents allow their children the space to discover and choose what they love, they're also allowing the athlete to guide the process. Physical activity is an important component of a healthy life, but as Meredith and her family realized, it doesn't have to come in the form of organized sports. It can also manifest in family hikes, a daily dog walk, or a game of tag in the backyard. Forcing competitive sports on children can result in burnout. When choosing sports, intrinsic motivation is important. When "becoming an athlete" is part of the family value system, you can never be sure that your child is choosing a sport because they love it or because they feel like it's just something they are required to do.

Often, caregivers forget to periodically check in with their children about what they want to do. Just because a child likes an activity one season doesn't necessarily mean they'll want to do it the next season, too. Whether they realize it or not, parents are always communicating. Your facial expressions, sighs, and tone of voice all send messages. If you tell a child they have a choice in their activities, your nonverbal communication has to match it, or they won't believe you. If you tell them they don't have to play hockey, dance, or swim if they don't want to, you want them to believe that their choice matters and is believed.

Angelina, for example, who competed for an NCAA Division I track and field team, remembers a time when she showed a lot of talent in swimming. Coaches and parents would tell her mom that she was a natural and had a lot of potential. However, in a conversation with her mom one day, she confessed that she didn't like being in the water— getting in the pool at 5:00 a.m. and 5:00 p.m. every day made her feel cold all the time. Her mom validated her feelings. "The fact that it was my choice was a positive," says Angelina, who's now an NCAA track and field coach. "I shared with my mom that I wanted to switch gears, and she allowed me to switch sports. She just matter-of-factly said that she respected that I didn't want to be cold."

Teens and young adults often say they wish they had tried more sports before they decided to specialize in just one. Adults and the youth sports system can make them feel like it's "too late" to try new activities, which is unfortunate. When families focus on a single sport, they invest in everything to make it happen. But sometimes when a young athlete is given the space, they choose a direction that the parent had not envisioned. Part of the process often requires letting go of your vision of the role sports would play in your family system or perhaps an underlying dream that your child may achieve your own athletic accomplishments that went unfulfilled. Maybe you love endurance sports, but your child wants to try figure skating. Perhaps you grew up in a soccer family and you wanted that same experience for your kids, but your daughter isn't interested. Grieving that loss is normal. In the end, giving your children the autonomy to make decisions that are best for them increases their connection to you.

You should also acknowledge that youth sports serve a purpose for adults, too, like friendships with other parents and a sense of community. Bonds are formed over the shared experience of athletics—traveling to weekend tournaments together, spending hours next to each other in the bleachers, coordinating carpools and dinners. If you give a young athlete the choice to try something else, you risk losing a group that you've also grown close to. And as a child shows improvement in a sport, parents also receive tangible feedback that their kid is doing something well, which can translate to feeling like you're also doing well as a parent. The validation can be intoxicating and boost the whole family's status within the sport's social ranks, too, even creating new opportunities and connections for parents outside of the team. It's hard to give it all up to let your child try something new.

It's okay to push children to honor their seasonal commitment (unless you've concluded it's a safety issue they're facing), but give them the option to try something else after they've fulfilled that obligation. Parents have a huge role to play in observing how their budding athletes respond to different environments and deciding if they need more or less of a challenge.

Chelsea Sodaro, the 2022 Ironman world champion, and her husband, who was also a collegiate track athlete, now have a daughter who is growing more active by the day. They have started thinking about how to handle her interest in sports when she's old enough to try them. "I know I don't want to coach her because I am intense and I don't want to put that on her," Chelsea says. "I want her to find purpose and meaning in life, but I don't want her to feel like her worth as a human being is based on her achievements. I don't want her to feel like that's where she's going to find her validation from her parents."

Indeed, we know that caregivers want sports to serve as a catalyst for young people to learn more about themselves and how they navigate the world around them. The less we put pressure on outcomes, the less likely children will compete from a place of fear and expectation, maximizing the opportunity that sports are giving them for character development and forming healthy habits.

Chapter Four

CREATING HEALTHY COACH-ATHLETE RELATIONSHIPS

A coach holds the most influence over every athlete's experience. Making sure that values and communication styles align is critical for mental health, longevity, and success.

Evelyn Gardner threw to home, and in the process, allowed the base runners to advance and blew a two-run lead for the Rockford Peaches of the All-American Girls Professional Baseball League. It was a big mistake, and her coach, Jimmy Dugan, berated her before she even made it to the dugout, screaming at her in front of her teammates, spectators, and the opposing team.

Evelyn, a quiet right fielder, dissolved into a puddle of tears.

"Are you crying? *Are you crying?*" Dugan yelled. "There's no crying! There's no crying in baseball!"

The umpire tossed Dugan out of the game for his obscenity-laden rage and the rest of the Rockford Peaches cheered the decision, happy to see their hot-tempered coach escorted from the field.

The scene was fictional, of course, bestowing one of the all-time best lines of the classic film, *A League of Their Own*. Sadly, it's also a scenario that many athletes can probably relate to, either having been the target of a coach's ire or observing it from a safe distance at some point in their sporting life. Tom Hanks, playing the disgruntled Coach Dugan, makes the situation humorous and oh-so-memorable, but we all realize it's less comical in real life. In today's world, most would call it verbal abuse with a healthy dose of bullying.

In the middle of his diatribe, Dugan confesses that when he was a baseball player, his manager yelled at him in much the same manner. His coaching approach had been handed down from generation to generation, with little thought to how it could have changed, evolved, or improved, especially for a new all-women's team. *A League of Their Own* was mostly a work of fiction, but parts of it still track. While many coaches would never dream of berating a player in this fashion, coaches sometimes default to the same "leadership" styles they were raised on, for better or worse, and often those strategies are based on the antiquated methods developed by men long ago and intended for male athletes. We know now that fear isn't a productive motivation tactic, no matter what your gender. Alas, we still see plenty of examples of intimidation by coaches in an effort to get results.

Like many NCAA athletes, Erika, a Division I swimmer, experienced a coaching turnover in her program and, when a new leader came in, she immediately noticed that his behavior was similar to that of her former youth club coach, which was triggering for her. He was quiet unless he was yelling, and any swimmers who weren't performing up to his expectations were invisible. When the team went to a training camp in Hawaii, the new coach refused to cancel practice even when the pool's chlorine pump malfunctioned. The water looked like milk, and the other groups who were using the facility decided against practice that day for safety reasons. Erika's coach demanded they get in the water. "Our suits were bleaching, goggle straps were snapping, and my eyebrows were pretty much gone," Erika says. "Other girls were bleeding."

After an hour, the coach told them to get out of the pool, but he demanded they make up the workout the next day, in addition to what was already on the schedule. "Some of my teammates told their parents what happened and they were livid," Erika says. "I begged my parents not to say anything because I didn't want one more thing to rock the boat—I didn't want him to have any more reason not to talk to me. He was already telling me I wasn't doing well and reminding me how much [scholarship] money they were giving me."

The coach-athlete relationship is the most important one in sport—the athlete depends on her coach for far more than game strategy and training plans, though that expertise is fundamental. The coach is also a mentor, motivator, consoler, counselor, teacher, and more. The best partnerships are based on trust. The athlete must have faith that the coach has her best interest and well-being at heart, that they share the same objectives, and that the coach believes in her. The coach must also trust the athlete to know herself best and make it safe for her to openly communicate what she's feeling. This kind of connection leads to mutual respect, shared goals, better performance, and greater perspective on what the team is trying to achieve, together and individually.

At the same time, by nature, the coach-athlete relationship has a vast power imbalance. The coach makes crucial decisions about what position athletes play, how much playing time they get, who advances to the next level (like the travel team), when they practice and for how long, and, for some athletes, colleges coaches eventually decide how much scholarship money they receive. Moreover, coaches control another valuable resource that athletes crave: praise and attention. One college swimmer named Emily told us how she felt ignored because she wasn't a top performer. One day while leaving the weight room, she crossed paths with the head coach. He tapped her on the shoulder and said, "Good job." She was shocked. "I texted my dad and it was a joke, but looking back, it's sad to me. I said, 'Wow, coach just told me "good job." Like, my career's complete. I finally got some praise from this head coach,'" Emily says. "It was funny to me at the time, but now it's sad when I think about it."

It becomes apparent why trust has to be the cornerstone of this bond and why the role of coach is complex and consuming, no matter what level or age group.

Caroline Doty, former assistant women's basketball coach at the University of Wisconsin, was a member of three national championship basketball teams at the University of Connecticut. She drew upon her experience as a former high-achieving player to guide seventeen athletes every year and has had ample opportunity to observe the different coaching philosophies and methods on the NCAA circuit. "The complexity of the role is not being their parent or their friend, but acknowledging that it involves critical moments of bonding," Caroline says.

Mary, a walk-on athlete for Wisconsin, remembers the days she struggled to go to practice. It was Caroline, who "was there with open arms and a big smile" who became a motivating force. "She was one call away, always, and every one of her players knew she cared about them," Mary says. "Because of that relationship she had with us, she could easily critique us and push us skill-wise because we knew we had built that trust and love with her beforehand."

In part, those connections were forged at Wisconsin through frequent individual meetings with the players to find out what was going on in their lives and how they were doing, not just on the court, but academically, socially, and otherwise. Understanding and nurturing the development of the whole person is essential. It's an opportunity to open the lines of communication and help athletes feel connected and supported. Time consuming? Yes. For coaches like Caroline Doty, practices, meetings, games, travel, recruiting, and more make coaching a round-the-clock endeavor. It becomes an identity for many in the profession, especially at the college level.

In fact, when the NCAA released a "Coach Well-Being" survey in January 2023,[1] it revealed that 40 percent of head coaches across all divisions feel "mentally exhausted" constantly or every day. They worry most about roster management and the evolving transfer landscape (providing more opportunities for athletes to switch schools), job security, budget cuts, and personal issues like finances and childcare. Others commented that the pressure to win while coping with budget cuts is a lot to handle. A Division III softball coach said, "Being on year-to-year contracts can be very concerning when so much of our job safety is in the hands of people eighteen to twenty-two years old . . . coaching while afraid of losing your job is a terrible way to feel."

All of this leaves one-third of college coaches feeling overwhelmed and experiencing sleep difficulties. Their number-one concern on the job, they said, is supporting student-athlete mental health; they ranked that issue higher than physical health, safety, athletic department gender equity, and inclusivity. "As coaches, the expectation is for us to be available for student-athlete crises 24/7," a Division II women's lacrosse coach reported, "while at the same time there is not consistent concern for our emotional and physical well-being."

It's a vicious cycle, isn't it? Athletes turn to their coaches for mental health support, but the coaches are pulled in so many directions, they need similar support themselves. And yet the system has so few protocols and policies in place, the problems persist.

Despite the exhaustion, coaches remain among the steadiest presences in young people's lives. But when tension, stress, and the pressure to win compound, the relationships can suffer. Caroline remained centered by remembering why she chose this path. "I want to give back to college athletes by giving them a great and ethical experience," she says. "When coaches fall out of alignment with why they chose to do this, there's an increase in abuse of power."

THE EARLY YEARS

Robert Hughes and Jay Coakley, who were sociologists at the University of Colorado, studied the "sport ethic" in a 1991 paper[2] that is still heavily referenced today. They found that athletes subscribe to a value system, or ethic, that includes sacrificing for their sport, playing through pain, accepting risks, and never accepting their limitations, to be considered (internally and externally) "real athletes." The sociologists point out that such conformity (or "overconforming" to these attributes, as they put it) can make athletes vulnerable. "Owners, managers, sponsors, and coaches—all of whom exercise control within the sport— often benefit when athletes over-accept and over-conform to the sport ethic," they wrote.

This ethic is embedded in sports, and yet when we examine it, it's evident that it doesn't help the athletes—and coaches have a responsibility to not allow it to drive their coaching.

From the beginning, young athletes should be introduced to what a healthy coaching situation looks and feels like. The problem isn't necessarily that coaches hold so much power but how they leverage, display, or communicate it. Our focus group of seven-year-olds, some of whom we introduced in chapters 1 and 2, have shared what they enjoy about their coaches from soccer, basketball, gymnastics, and other sports they're eagerly exploring. Molly, for example, says her favorite part of practice is when her coach braids her hair. We imagine that Molly likes the special one-on-one time that such an activity affords. Bowen notices that her coaches "feel proud when we score." And Rian likes that her coaches say, "When we lose, we are learning something for next time." Everly is a keen observer of the "coach's kid," who she thinks is the best player on the team because, "the coach always takes his time to look at her, and she always knows what to do because her dad is the coach." An important lesson for coaches, courtesy of budding basketball star Everly: they're always watching you, and they pick up on much more than you realize.

From these brief accounts, it seems our group of first and second graders have landed in youth sport programs that likely have the priorities in check. It's challenging for coaches to keep girls engaged at this age, while they're progressing and developing at different rates; juggling the interest and ability levels is no easy task. Up until age twelve, the best way to guide them is to allow them to discover and explore sports on their own terms. Coaches should merely provide enjoyable ways to introduce motor skills (like playing in an open gym or on the field), learn basic rules that are transferable between sports, and emphasize practice over performance. At this stage, budding athletes are hopefully discovering that physical movement combined with community and friendship is something they enjoy and want to do, in some form, for the rest of their lives.

Ally, a gymnast who went on to compete in college, remembers the big whiteboard the coaches put in the gym when she was just starting out as a child. It displayed an inspiring quote of the week and gave team members a space to share how they were feeling that day. The team was encouraged to participate in weekly check-ins with their coaches and the rest of the group, which was a way to bond as a team. Every Saturday practice started with learning a new dance together—a time she remembers as silly and fun before more serious training began. Ally could already put a lot of pressure on herself back then, and her coaches worked hard to help her enjoy the sport. "I liked competition because I took the sport seriously," Ally says. "At one meet, I remember my coaches on the sidelines making bird noises at me so that I would smile. They helped us keep perspective."

In 2019, the Women's Sports Foundation commissioned a comprehensive study, "Coaching Through a Gendered Lens: Maximizing Girls' Play and Potential,"[3] which examined the intersection of girls' development with coaching practices in an effort to understand the factors that lead to female participation and persistence in sport. The foundation wanted a better understanding of the coaching practices that can overcome some of the common barriers to keeping girls active and engaged. The research included interviews with experts in girls' sport, a national survey of 1,129 girls between the ages of seven to thirteen who participate in sports, their parents, and a sample of sixty-four programs identified by the Women's Sports Foundation as "exemplary" for providing quality sports opportunities to underserved girls.

The key findings? Girls loved programs that emphasized social interaction, had coaches that they liked, and offered an environment where they could try new skills without facing repercussions for failure. Coaches directly influenced whether girls intended to keep playing; the coaches who fostered supportive relationships and used a mastery-based approach, meaning goals and rewards were focused on improving skills, were preferred. Girls wanted coaches to keep things fun, but also enjoyed healthy competition. In fact, they indicated that competition and winning were a big part of what made sports fun, as long as they weren't afraid to make mistakes or fall short in the process.

Based on those survey results, the experts recommend meeting the girls' interest in competition while also providing a great social experience. Those objectives aren't mutually exclusive. Eliminating competition, the experts warned, "sends a message that their sport involvement is not taken as seriously [as boys] . . . which can result in girls' lower perceived competence and sense of belonging." As another expert noted in the Women's Sports Foundation report: "You don't have to be soft, just nice. Do not infantilize or underestimate girls' ability. Treat girls as powerful, strong, very capable individuals."

Kids know what they want and need, if only adults would listen to them. Among the athletes that Harry Marra has coached is Brianne Eaton, a now retired heptathlete who won multiple world and Olympic medals during her decorated career. As a highly successful elite coach, Harry's advice to youth coaches is to keep it simple and to "cultivate the keen senses that kids already have." He can give multiple examples of why he believes kids are born doing most of the mechanics of sport correctly and why skills are innate to them. He shows videos of a young girl with no training perfectly executing long-jump form, for instance. But too often, it's the coaches and parents who inadvertently train or teach those instincts out of them, leading young athletes to question what they probably already know, he says.

Harry implores athletes—even those at the most elite level, like Brianne—to connect to their natural instincts. After all he's seen and experienced, he has concluded that what interferes with their ability to do that is that the system of athletics we've created in the United States at every level has been complicated with power and money (earned by winning, sometimes at all costs). He's guided the careers of the world's best, and in the process has refused the distraction. All he wants is for athletes to progress to the next stage of life feeling like empowered people who trust themselves to know what they need to lead happy, fulfilling lives.

"While we were very focused on a singular athletic goal—winning an Olympic gold medal—there was never a time when I felt he put that as a higher priority than our mental and physical well-being," says Brianne, whose husband, double gold medalist decathlete Ashton Eaton, was also coached by Harry. "[The approach] encouraged us to take a total break from training and competition for three months of the year, which is unheard of as track and field athletes. We quickly learned just how important it was to travel for leisure, visit our families, and enjoy extracurricular activities we wouldn't otherwise be able to do."

Moral of the story? Listen to young athletes. If girls are asking to compete, for example, coaches should learn how to create safe, fun-focused spaces for them to do so. Let them win and let them lose—and treat each situation with positive reinforcement. Neither victory nor defeat at this point should come with punishment or reward. Receptive coaches should observe the team's weaknesses and integrate new drills and skills at practice but not shame the team for what it got wrong. Everything is a growth opportunity. It's all about building belief, confidence, and work ethic in athletes, not about the actual victory. Remember the Olympic creed: "The important thing in life is not the triumph, but the fight; the essential thing is not to have won, but to have fought well."

Parents looking for signs that their children feel supported by their coach and are enjoying the process should take notice of their behaviors. Are they excited to go to practice? Do they talk about wanting more playing time? Do they share stories about games and practices? How do they sound when they talk about their experiences—animated and excited or deflated and frustrated? Do they initiate practicing at home? All of these are indicators that they're finding fulfillment in the activity. If they begin to show other consistent behaviors like belly aches, body pains, or irritability when it's time to head to practice, then check in and ask if there's something they aren't enjoying about the experience or if something about their coach may be rubbing them the wrong way. While we'll dig deeper into sexual, emotional, and verbal abuse in chapter 6, it's important to recognize the host of red flags that should make athletes and parents seek out different arrangements (and, probably, report the inappropriate behavior to officials, whether at the US Center for SafeSport, a Title IX officer, or the sport's governing body, who can investigate it). Some call it "tough coaching," and while there's room for a coach who demands discipline and has high expectations, when it crosses the line into manipulation and bullying, which often results in depression, anxiety, or other mental health conditions, it's no longer an acceptable coaching practice.

TRAINING FOR COACHES

Among the challenges for coaches is finding guidance on how to cultivate healthy relationships and expectations with their athletes. While certifications and credentialing programs exist for every sport, many are not mandated, and often the only requirement to become a coach is passing a criminal background check. Even so, according to the Aspen Institute's 2022 Project Play report,[4] 45 percent of unpaid coaches were more likely than paid coaches to never receive evaluations. These coaches expressed less confidence in a variety of areas, including helping athletes succeed academically, setting clear expectations for how the coach chooses a team, teaching skills, maximizing team strengths during competition, assessing physical conditioning, and identifying mental health challenges.

Even paid coaches—whether at the youth, collegiate, or professional levels—often don't receive more formalized training, which is troubling given how much influence they have with young people. Still fewer opportunities are available for them to learn to guide the athletic pursuits of girls and women, specifically, who have different physiology and psychology than boys and men. It can lead to troubling circumstances for coaches and athletes; if the only metric we're measuring is their win-loss record, it leaves little incentive to focus on other significant factors that are in the long-term best interests of players. Are athletes pressured to perform even in the throes of illness or injury, for example? What ensures that coaches remain ethical if their only measurable outcome is winning? Don't get us wrong. Winning is important and it should be recognized and rewarded. But *how* a coach wins is also paramount, and Jimmy Dugan–style is not it.

Victoria, a track and cross-country athlete at a southern Division I university, started her collegiate career with an emotionally unstable coach who regularly screamed at the women during practice. "She threatened us on a regular basis that if we didn't perform better, she'd lose her job and we'd lose our scholarships," she says. "That was her coaching style." Fortunately, the coach was indeed fired, and the new staff routinely asks how Victoria and her teammates are doing. They also consistently offer affirmation of her progress. "They ask us all the time if there's anything going on that would make it difficult to perform that day," she says. That simple, open-ended question results in a culture of trust and allows team members to be more transparent about their physical and mental well-being.

Sade*, a triathlete and swimmer at a college in the Midwest, says her coaches treat their team members "like real people" and encourage all of them to go to therapy, even if a therapist is just providing one more space to talk. "If we have large assignments due that we're stressed about, we don't have to swim so we can take that extra time and put it toward work," Sade says, adding that the coaches take away racing opportunities if grades are declining.

Taking an active interest in the mental well-being of athletes is an aspect of coaching that's becoming more recognized—and it's a tall order. While coaches know that they are often acting as mental health first responders, they aren't typically given the proper training to know exactly what that means or what protocols to follow should they discover that an athlete is suffering from a condition like an eating disorder, anxiety, depression, self-harm, or suicidal thoughts. The NCAA offers universities comprehensive best practices for providing mental health care but only requires Division I institutions to provide mental health services to athletes, which doesn't account for long wait times or insufficient licensed staffing. With a nationwide shortage in mental-health care providers, it's difficult for coaches to ensure that their teams are getting what they need. More than one athlete told us that they felt like their privacy was violated by the athletic department's mental health provider, who'd share stories from teammates or tell coaches what they heard in sessions that were meant to remain confidential.

It's a different landscape than even ten years ago, when a coach wouldn't dare ask an athlete about suicidal thoughts. The increased awareness about mental health is encouraging, but coaches also need the tools to turn that awareness into the appropriate action. We talked to one coach who insisted that an athlete go to the emergency room, after she shared that she had suicidal thoughts. He didn't know at the time that suicide exists on a spectrum and that some people live with chronic thoughts of dying, and he was appalled when the ER discharged the athlete, doubting that the ER properly evaluated the athlete. So, he asked the athlete to return home to receive care, instead of relying on a mental health professional's advice (which he may not have had access to). The athlete never attempted suicide, didn't return to campus, and was stripped of her place of belonging.

If we were to speculate, the coach unknowingly removed this person's "protective factor," which is an aspect of life that helps a person with suicidal thoughts gain perspective on what matters to them. A protective factor minimizes the risk of acting on these suicidal thoughts—it motivates them to stay alive. Often, it can be a place on a team, and taking it away can sometimes do more harm than good. But the coach and staff can't know these intricacies of mental health without any education on what to look for and how to communicate with an athlete who they suspect is suffering. There they are on the front lines, the adults who players see and talk to most consistently, but they are often without the basic training that could provide a lifeline. In this case, the coach was driven by fear. That fear, combined with a lack of training, led him to a harmful decision. Instead, the coach should have been able to rely on mental health professionals and medical staff to guide the athlete's path forward.

Kailani, the track athlete competing for a small university in Texas, turned to her coach when she didn't know who else to talk to about her intense depression as she was coping with a challenging transition to college life. The coach at the time was dismissive and told Kailani that help was not available to her on campus, so she struggled alone with nobody to talk to. "I had a racing mind, poor appetite and sleep schedule, little to no energy, and I was either overly emotional or not emotional at all," she says. The following semester, a new coach took over the program and reached out to Kailani, wanting to know what she was going through and what had happened the previous year. "It was a game changer," she says. "He offered so much positive reinforcement and helped me find a safe place in running again." All the coach did was validate her feelings and experience and follow that up with support.

Quality coaches, according to the US Olympic and Paralympic Committee's coaching education,[5] are interested in holistic development, which includes concern about personal, emotional, cultural, and social identity. Coaches and athletes should jointly set challenging goals in line with age and ability, and coaches should provide rationale for decisions, recognition of progress, and account for factors outside of sport that may affect training and performance.

For example, a collegiate acrobatics and tumbling team welcomed a first-year student from a rural area to the squad. The only reason her geographic background is important is because it was used to excuse her racist behavior—as if she didn't know better because of where she came from. During the first weeks on campus, while members of the team were gathered in a dorm room, she suggested that during a song that included the N-word in the chorus, the group point toward their Black teammates. The athlete thought it would be funny, even after a Black team member explained that it was racist and offensive. She did it anyway, and the coaches didn't intervene effectively after it was reported to them. The university's administration got involved and sent a staff person of color to speak to the team, although this employee was not trained to facilitate this kind of intervention or provide team support. The message to the group was that the young, white athlete from a small town didn't understand and it was *their* job to teach her, instead of acknowledging the harm and to give support to those who felt it. This is a common problem: institutions often attend to white perpetrators instead of the ways that racism permeates the system. None of the coaches had the tools to step in and instead made the Black athletes feel as though it was their responsibility to "be the bigger people."

Ultimately, the white athlete left the team, and it allowed those who were harmed to heal. The athletes were still concerned about the impact of the situation on mental health, as well as their general sense of safety, but when they asked the coach, who was white, to address what had happened, she was restricted by the administration from talking about it. One of the basic agreed-upon values on any team should be that racism in any form won't be tolerated, and that message should come from the top. To build general trust, the coach would need to clearly articulate how the group will avoid such scenarios in the future and how athletes will be better supported if problems arise. The system has a responsibility to uplift and protect the marginalized.

We asked a lot of coaches about the litany of responsibilities that end up under their purview. In the most underfunded programs, they're the go-to for every need. They act as counselors, nutritionists, physical therapists, friends, parental figures, DEI (diversity, equity, and inclusion) directors, travel agents, and, yes, coaches, yet they can't possibly embody all these roles. They must know where their expertise and experience begin and end and where to find education or support when the need is outside their realm. In the case of antibias training, more resources are available, like RISE, a curriculum designed to educate the sports community on racial discrimination and championing social justice; or A Long Talk, which offers anti-racism workshops in sports settings. The US Soccer Foundation partners with Mom of All Capes, which provides an anti-racist coaching toolkit.

Coaches who have higher emotional intelligence and greater awareness of their own emotions are the ones who are most capable of providing a safe and successful experience. They are less defensive, less reactionary, and even-keeled. And they can help their athletes regulate those inevitable emotional fluctuations as well. Just like the parents and caregivers, coaches foster a healthier and more ethical culture when they aren't white-knuckling their way through games and seasons and keep their verbal and nonverbal communication consistent and in check, remembering that their tone of voice and facial expressions can lead an athlete to either give up or show up. The coaches who continue to learn, grow, pivot, and evolve—and who are willing to make their own mistakes and also admit them—are the ones who ultimately achieve their goals and those of the teams they lead.

RECOGNIZING RED FLAGS AND HONORING BOUNDARIES

Emily started swimming at age seven, and her dream came true when she got a scholarship to a Power Five D-I program in the south. She had always wanted to go to a university with a big football team and a lot of school spirit, and it seemed like it was all coming together. But when she attended her first practices with the head coach, it immediately felt "weird." He separated the first-year swimmers from the rest of the team, handed them sponges, and demanded that they scrub the starting blocks. "The feeling and the vibe was [that] we were at the bottom and we needed to work our way up by volunteering for grunt work tasks," Emily says. "It was a seniority-based team, which was hard."

Soon she realized that team members would get in trouble for what they did on the weekends, but instead of disciplining those individuals, the coaches would yell at the entire group. Once, some underaged swimmers had hopped a fence to gain entry into a bar. When the coaches found out, they opted to shame the transgressors instead of going through normal disciplinary channels: the swimmers were told to flip their apparel and swim caps inside out because they didn't deserve the privilege of wearing the school's logo anymore. The coach reprimanded swimmers for being late if they weren't fifteen minutes early for practice, not in an effort to instill punctuality as a life skill but to add an element of rigidity and another fear tactic. To make sure she never got in trouble, Emily would arrive forty-five minutes before start time. Her anxiety soon escalated to the point where she struggled to eat enough to fuel her training. The coaches were erratic and unpredictable, which underpinned the entire team culture. While the men's team could get away with a lot of crude, horrific behavior, the women were given no margin for error. The sport she had loved since she was a child now only made Emily sick with worry. "I felt this constant humming. My heart rate was elevated, and it was unsettling," she recalls.

Athletes should be held accountable for bad behavior, of course, but it's on coaches to make expectations and consequences clear and consistent and communicate them in ways that make sense to the athletes. Some accomplish this with team agreements that specifically outline what is expected from everybody who participates and can include factors like academic standards, behavior policies, commitment to training, and teamwork. We recommend that team members be involved in creating team agreements, especially on women's teams, where sometimes athletes seem to be held to higher standards of behavior than, say, the football players who, on many campuses, might get away with behavior that others wouldn't. Giving athletes input on the agreement can increase buy-in and create transparency. And it should include clauses regarding what team members can expect from their coaches, who should promise to treat each athlete fairly and respectfully.

The boundaries of what constitutes acceptable behavior for coaches shift as athletes get older. For example, coaches should never communicate with young athletes individually through text, email, or social media—either the entire team should be included, or parents copied, or both—neither should young athletes ever find themselves in a one-on-one transportation situation with the coach.

Coaches who seek to tightly control athletes' lives outside of training, like limiting time with family, friends, and significant others, or even seeking too much information about an athlete's dating life, are crossing a line and could be trying to isolate the athlete from her support network. Other examples of emotional misconduct include stalking athletes on social media, ignoring an athlete for extended periods of time and/or excluding her from practice, and taunting, name-calling, humiliating, intimidating, or threatening a player. Commenting on physical appearance in any way—especially body-shaming—is also inappropriate and harmful.

But the truth is, fear-based coaching isn't just harmful; it doesn't produce results, either. It conditions athletes to want to perform only to survive or avoid ridicule; they're trying to please an authority figure who has all the decision-making power, instead of working as a team and achieving objectives together. "Tough" coaching may work in the short-term, but it will never produce long-term success. And it causes damage to the athletes' well-being that may take years to treat.

Sport systems should also do more to evaluate how coaches achieve those winning records and incentivize them to also do so ethically. Some other metrics that could foster improved athlete well-being: percentage of athletes who complete their eligibility (the allotted years that a college athlete is allowed to compete), bone injury or overuse injury rates, ratio of team alumni who donate to the program, and athlete evaluations, for example.

DIVERSIFY THE COACHING POOL

It's no surprise that most sports are led by white men. All the statistics back up the observation you can plainly see for yourself on television, social media, or the sports section of the local newspaper. The Tucker Center for Research on Girls & Women in Sport issues a "report card" each year,[6] detailing how many NCAA women's teams are led by women and women of color. In 2021, the NCAA had a total of 3,617 head coaches of women's teams from 357 Division I institutions. Of those, women held 42.7 percent of head coaching roles, while female coaches of color represented just 7.3 percent of head coaches of women's teams. In the 2022 report, based on a sample of 980 head coach positions of women's NCAA teams from eighty-seven institutions, the overall percentage of women's teams with women head coaches was 46 percent, which marked a 2.3 percent increase from the prior year. Note, however, that women still held less than half of the head coaching positions for women's teams.

At the youth level, according to the Aspen Institute's Project Play report, women comprise only 26 percent of adults coaching kids fourteen and under, despite the growth in female sports participation. Men are twice as likely to coach girls in youth sports as women are likely to coach boys, illustrating the ongoing bias associated with women coaching male athletes at all levels of sport.

While other industries have made progress in parity among leadership, it seems coaching has remained stagnant. You may wonder why it matters, but it matters a lot for female athletes. It's not that men can't or shouldn't coach women—of course they can and should—but in any sector, when most of the population is left out of the room, the organization will lack critical skills, perspectives, and expertise that lead to achieving goals (in this case, winning). Coaching is no different.

We know that female coaches in girls' sports serve as role models and shift the perception that sport is not meant for girls. Seeing women, and especially women of color, in leadership positions gives girls a greater understanding of their potential and counters all the stereotypes that they see in sports. They are also more likely to open up to a female coach about issues like body image, puberty, and periods—essential topics on which girls need guidance from trusted adults, and ones who, without education and empathy, take girls out of sport for good (we'll cover all of them in depth in the next few chapters).

Many girls told us that when they speak openly about their periods, for example, with their male coaches, they can sense their coaches' discomfort. "The male coach would say, 'Just tell me when you get your period and we will adjust the workout,'" says Camille, a high school cross-country runner in the Pacific Northwest. "But he didn't actually know anything about running and being on your period. Our female coach researches cycles and the impact on the female body and training." Camille says she's learned much more about RED-S and why it's important for women's health to make sure that their energy intake matches their output from her female coaches than from her male coaches.

According to the Women's Sports Foundation,[7] young female athletes are "more likely to believe a female coach's advice because they've lived it." In its survey, girls who said they "really" or "really, really like their coach a lot" were more likely to have a female coach (82 percent vs. 73 percent) than girls who said they liked their coach "a little" or "don't like them at all."

The career path is daunting for women, especially at the collegiate level, where white men are usually doing the hiring—just 25 percent of NCAA athletic directors are female[8]—and so often feel more comfortable hiring the other men they know or who look like them. As a result, women often take low-paying assistant coaching positions that have no opportunity for advancement. To move to the next level, they often have to relocate, which makes family life and childcare difficult to manage.

Female coaches also tend to be evaluated more harshly than their male counterparts. Tara, for example, was a women's soccer coach at a large Division I program in the Pacific Northwest and was highly celebrated when her team won, but when she showed up at the department staff meeting after a loss, she "felt like 'loser' was plastered on my forehead." Her worth was completely based on wins, and she was constantly treated differently depending on the outcome of games. In her seventh season, the cards were laid out for her by the administration—if the team didn't produce the desired results, she'd be fired. She was friends with the men's basketball and football coaches who shrugged it off, saying, "It's no big deal. Everyone gets fired." One of them had been fired five times. "But men's salaries can absorb a move, a risk, or a layoff. My salary would not support that," Tara says. "The risk was too high to just move all over the country with two young kids. I didn't hit my marks that season and was immediately let go. The inequity of pay for women forces you out of the profession."

It's a combination of pay disparity and mistreatment that drive so many female coaches out of the profession. Women are working in overdrive just to prove they are qualified, and they sometimes absorb that extra hustle as just part of the job. Equal pay is a tangible talking point, though. Female coaches can't always find trustworthy advocates to talk to about mistreatment, but pointing to indisputable numbers on a pay scale can sometimes feel easier.

Despite these challenges, for women like Rhonda Riley, who played soccer and ran track in high school and became a volunteer coach at a high school track program while attending Oregon State University, coaching can be a uniquely rewarding experience. She went on runs with the team, bonded with the girls, and enjoyed getting to know them as athletes and people. She loved the role that she played in their lives, mentoring and teaching while moving and engaging in a shared favorite activity. After she graduated, Oregon State University started a women's track and field and cross-country program. Rhonda walked into the head coach's office and told him how she fell in love with coaching and described what she could offer the new team. He offered her a volunteer position and she took it. As she solidified her belief that coaching was her professional path, she enrolled at Arizona State to pursue a graduate degree in education leadership and serve as the track and field graduate assistant coach. While she was there, the team won two national titles and she gained experience and knowledge in how top programs operate, eventually becoming the director of operations and managing the budget, logistics, and schedules.

When she finished her master's program, Rhonda moved on again, this time to another assistant coaching role at Vanderbilt. She stayed in that position for nine years—a long time for an assistant coach. But she found that she enjoyed working with the head coach and the team had steadily improved during her tenure, finishing sixth at the national championships during her fourth year. By 2016, Duke University called and offered Rhonda the role of head coach of women's distance running. The head coach at Vanderbilt suggested that she take it; she had reached her ceiling at Vanderbilt.

Up until 2020, Rhonda spearheaded a lot of success for the Duke distance squad. But then, around the time when the pandemic started, the director of the program decided to retire, and Rhonda became the interim cross-country head coach. She started working with the men's team, too, and connected with the new athletes who were entering a big life transition at a precarious time. To this day, she still gets texts from track and field athletes who appreciated how much she cared for them. Rhonda applied for the permanent position of director, but the program offered it to somebody else. Though she was disappointed, it offered her an opportunity to evaluate the direction of her career and how she could best align it with her values—keeping athletes' health and well-being at the forefront, even if that didn't always mean a team would win.

Rhonda reports she's now the happiest she's ever been, working in real estate and taking on a volunteer coaching role at Portland State University. She gets to do exactly what she loves—motivating, inspiring, and mentoring in a culture that supports her style. She continues to direct a women-in-coaching organization geared toward supporting female coaches. The group is striving to retain the youngest coaches in their twenties and thirties to ensure the landscape of sport shifts as the men who have held leadership positions for generations, now in their seventies, retire. "They have, for decades, set the tone and culture of the sport," Rhonda says. "Change is on the horizon."

Chapter Five

PUBERTY, PERIODS, AND PLAYING
SPORTS

Adolescence is rife with physical and psychological
challenges for active girls. Without support and education
from caregivers, peers, and coaches, they often
struggle with body image.

It seems that right around the time families have settled into routines
and have gotten a grasp on how to integrate sports into their lives,
their daughters reach the age of puberty, and everything is turned
upside down. If it feels that way to parents and caregivers, just imagine
how much upheaval the girls themselves are experiencing physically
and emotionally, internally and externally—straddling life as a child
while emerging as a young adult. The preteen and teen years are a significant turning point for female athletes and a chapter that can have
long-term implications. Just ask Leslie Lu, now a twenty-one-year-old
volleyball player at a mid-Atlantic NCAA Division III institution,
whose life today is deeply tied to her preteen development.

By fourth grade, Leslie Lu already stood at five foot five, towering
over her entire class. At the time, her stature was a point of pride. It

was praised in dance, where her long legs and slim figure were admired. And in early middle school, her physique made her a natural to try out for the volleyball team. "Many girls were jealous of me. I bonded with my coach because I had never had someone see potential in me in a sport," Leslie Lu remembers. But soon, Leslie Lu's body hit adolescence and puberty. Around age twelve, she was one of the first in her peer group to get her period and nothing about it felt "normal" to her. "I felt alone, depressed, and anxious," Leslie Lu says. "And when it came to sports, I was judged in the locker room because they could hear the wrapper of my pads and tampons. I was terrified to bend over or fall down. Girls were so brutal to me, and the boys would snicker if they had even the slightest information about that time of the month."

By her first year of high school, Leslie Lu was diagnosed with an eating disorder. As she developed more quickly than the others in her dance classes, she felt like the "big girl," so she pushed herself to run every day, in addition to playing volleyball and soccer, and started using a calorie tracker and restricting herself to a vegetarian diet to lose weight. "I was scared of my body getting bigger . . . I didn't want to disappoint my dance teacher or my coaches," Leslie Lu says. "I needed to be in my best shape, and it ultimately turned me into a bag of bones."

In college, Leslie Lu has remained scared of gaining muscle even though her muscle development contributes to her strength on the court and reduces injury risks. When the number on the scale climbs, she compensates by eating less. She's only had her period ten times in four years, a symptom of RED-S (which, as a reminder, is a syndrome of health risks when athletes' caloric intake is deficient in supporting their energy demands). Yet, she says, doctors haven't indicated during her physicals that her amenorrhea (missed period) is a sign of any larger health problems. "College athletics have pushed my body to an extreme place," Leslie Lu says. "My body and I have a love-hate relationship.

There are days where I am extremely happy to be in my skin, but other days I wish I could just crawl out of it. I still go through days of not eating, and then binging within the next few."

Leslie Lu's story is common among countless girls and women in sport. Puberty is one of the most challenging transitions they'll face, yet it's also among the least talked about. The lack of education to prepare girls for the ways their bodies will grow and change leads to these preventable outcomes like confusion, humiliation, and frustration (at best), or injuries, body image and eating disorders, RED-S, and other long-term health risks (at worst). Puberty occurs at different times for everybody, but the process is linear in the absence of interventions like puberty blockers.

These rapid physical and hormonal shifts come just as girls are also facing increased pressure to perform, new social landscapes, and more rigorous academic demands. Then there's that myth that lingers in sports culture even today: that puberty and menstruation will lead to performance declines—that their days of excelling on the playing field are over for good. On the whole, our culture does not adequately inform girls (and the people still feeding them these lies) that the growth and maturity they're going through is actually a sign of health and strength. Historically, there's been a lack of research about how to successfully coach female athletes through these adolescent and young adult years, which leaves little mystery about why so many of them decide to quit sports by age fourteen. They watch boys gain muscle mass, while getting stronger and faster. Meanwhile, girls may gain up to twenty-three pounds while their bodies are growing and preparing for menstruation. In fact, according to the American Academy of Pediatrics, about 25 percent of growth in height occurs during puberty.[1] They hit temporary performance plateaus, finding it awkward to move bodies that now include hips and breasts, and may have a temporary reduction in aerobic capacity and strength. But it will pass. They'll learn how to function and thrive as athletes as they reestablish their centers of gravity, balance, and body control.

PREPARING AND PATIENCE

How coaches and parents prepare girls for what's happening can make a difference in how they cope during puberty, which typically starts between ages eight and thirteen. Explaining what they're going to experience, normalizing it, and allowing them to have conversations about it among themselves and with trusted adults help make the discussion of puberty and periods less taboo. Reassurance and knowledge that what they are going through is perfectly normal are necessary for keeping girls healthy and active.

In fact, the world's first suicide prevention hotline was established after a fourteen-year-old girl in England died by suicide in 1935 after she started menstruating for the first time.[2] She was never told about puberty or periods, so she thought something was wrong with her. With nobody to talk to, she made a desperate choice to die. In turn, Chad Varah, the priest who officiated her burial, vowed to educate people about sexual health. He inspired what became known as the Samaritans, an international suicide prevention and mental health services organization. Varah believed that people experiencing suicidal thoughts often just needed to talk to somebody who could offer kindness, patience, and advice.

The philosophy holds true today when it comes to coping with the onset of puberty. Sara Hall, one of the fastest American marathon runners of all-time, finished fifth in the 2022 World Championships, at age thirty-nine. As a girl growing up in Northern California, she played soccer for many years before deciding to focus on running. She remembers, before her senior year in high school, she went to Europe for the summer, putting training mostly on hold until she returned to cross-country season in the fall. Her body had changed while she was away. She had "curves" for the first time. Also, for the first time, her performance wasn't improving, and in some cases, her times were slower. But Sara credits her coach for getting her through it, helping her see that the performance plateaus were only temporary by incrementally building her training back up, as well as encouraging rest and recovery, along with healthy, nourishing fueling habits. "I finished the season winning the Foot Locker Championships," Sara says. "Even though my body had retained that weight, I was learning to be stronger and grow into it."

Counter Sara's progression with that of a thirteen-year-old girl in the northwest who had shown promise in cycling but had fallen into binging and hiding food in her bedroom. Her parents were strict about providing healthy food for their daughter and son, and they didn't allow candy, chips, or "junk" in the house. The girl's mom, who had also been a cyclist, attributed her own success to her nutrition and believed that her daughter had "real potential" if only she could "get a grasp on her eating and body weight." The mom restricted her daughter's diet believing if she could have more control over the food she consumed, she'd mitigate the effects of puberty and remain a successful athlete. It resulted in her daughter's disordered eating, decreased self-esteem, and onset of anxiety. The daughter had difficulty navigating daily living because this controlling parenting style hadn't given her the space to develop her own intuition or decision-making skills.

Parents, caregivers, and coaches all hand down their experiences to the next generation whether they realize it or not—and whether it's as overt as a mother who controls her daughter's diet to improve athletic performance during puberty. To be sure, any trauma that adults had experienced during their own puberty has stuck with them, and it can influence how their kids view themselves, too. Members of our parent focus group recalled the fears, embarrassment, and shame they felt when they first got their periods. Women in the group confessed that they began criticizing their bodies around that time in their lives, and many have never stopped. Although they don't want their daughters to fall into the same body image traps, it's fair to speculate that their children notice all the ways in which their actions say otherwise. Dieting, bemoaning the shape of their thighs or their lack of abs, cosmetic surgery, shapewear, and more reinforce the belief that smaller will always be better.

Adults can break these cycles, however. Ellen*, an educator and mother of two in the Pacific Northwest, including a twelve-year-old daughter, has tried to create a home, alongside her partner, that values transparency, curiosity, and conversation. One topic they talk about a lot is periods, in preparation for her daughter's first one. They've bought period underwear, a book about puberty, and Ellen has talked openly about her own cycle, so her daughter understands what to expect. She doesn't want her to cry, like she did, the first time she menstruates. They've created a "period pack" to put in her daughter's bag, containing all the products like underwear, pads, and tampons, that she will need when the time comes, and explained the purpose of each and how to use them. "I'm creating a different experience than the one I had," Ellen says. "Despite the best of intentions, my parents didn't talk about puberty, and I was somewhat ashamed as my body began to change."

In fact, Ellen's home has become a place where body-shaming of any kind is unacceptable, including self-criticism. They don't label foods "good" or "bad," either—it's all food and it all serves a different purpose, most importantly as fuel. "As a generation of women who, at a minimum, were raised at a time when bodies were regularly commented on and the narrative around weight and image were deeply ingrained, we know that our daughters are always listening and observing," Ellen says. "The work to override that conditioning is critical."

Ellen's daughter hasn't specialized in a particular sport yet, but she enjoys dance, travel soccer, swim team, and community basketball. Mostly, the family emphasizes sports as a healthy activity that cultivates a sense of belonging and social connection. At a recent dinner party, the parents were sitting at one table eavesdropping on their daughters at another table, and they overheard a conversation about periods, body changes, and how one girl's mom helped her shave her armpits. It was satisfying to discover that these girls have become so much more comfortable discussing what they're going through and sharing the strategies that have been helpful. After all, they see each other in the hallways at school, on the playing fields, and especially in the locker rooms.

Having each other's backs is comforting and confidence-boosting, especially as they're entering their teen years.

STAYING ACTIVE

Girls need all the support they can get during this stage. While all these rapid physical changes are taking place, their brains are also changing quickly. At this point, for example, they may fail to connect how regular training and practice lead to athletic success, believing that failure or accomplishment are due to their own unique talent or lack of talent. Or they may not understand that the lack of control over their changing bodies may cause a feeling of less control over other aspects of life. They often become frustrated because at this time of life, they're also temporarily more susceptible to injuries as their centers of gravity shift.

This is also a time when girls may experience symptoms of anxiety, depression, attention deficit disorder, and self-harm. Life can generally feel more stressful to teens, but hormonal changes associated with puberty may also play a role. According to the US Office on Women's Health, changing levels of estrogen and progesterone during the menstrual cycle can cause symptoms of depression and anxiety. It's a difficult period for caregivers and coaches to differentiate between normal mood swings and more serious mental health issues.

We also can't discount the fact that young female athletes are often led to believe that their progress and trajectory in sports will be linear, so when this temporary plateau hits, just as they are navigating all the rapid changes in their bodies and the upheaval of moods and emotions, stagnant performance can undermine their confidence, self-worth, and connection to self, and they are not always given the support or guidance they need to get through it. In fact, in some documented cases in gymnastics and figure skating, they've been encouraged to stunt their physical development to remain competitive under the belief that smaller is better.

Cat, who competed at the world level in swimming before she started college, remembers how swimmers celebrated those who developed later—at sixteen instead of thirteen, for example. In fact, coaches pushed girls to try to delay their periods, often through restrictive eating and/or excessive exercise. She may have been one of them. "I guarantee if I had not been training so hard, I would have gone through puberty sooner," Cat says, admitting that after menstruating four times, she didn't get her period for two years. "Doctors would ask me when my last period was and I'd say, 'Two years ago,' and they'd just say, 'Oh, that's because you're an athlete.'"

During those teenage years, Cat says her male coaches just held the girls to the same standards as the boys, refusing to acknowledge the biological differences going on. "Guys could be consistent and girls would be more inconsistent, and there was no tolerance for that," she says. In retrospect, she now knows that peaks in performance come and go regardless of hormonal changes. "You drop less time when you are older than when you are still growing," she says. "There is a science that isn't controllable."

Sade, a triathlete at a Midwestern Division III program, was also coached by men during high school sports, including track and field. Back then she remembers coaches and athletic trainers who didn't understand that when girls weren't getting their periods, they were likely experiencing RED-S, which, as we've already discussed, leads to a host of health problems for still-growing teens, as well as a decline in athletic performance. Now at the collegiate level, Sade says her two female coaches are sticklers for proper fueling. "In high school, the coaches said, 'It's fine. You're a distance runner. It's okay you're not getting your period,'" she says. "But in college they tell us to go to our athletic trainer and a doctor and make sure we're eating enough. For a lot of us, it's the first time anybody said anything like that to us."

Decorated US track star Lauren Fleshman, who wrote the memoir *Good for a Girl: A Woman Running in a Man's World*, first penned "Dear Younger Me,"[3] in a 2017 column that appeared on MileSplit, a website geared toward youth track and field athletes, warning girls following in her footsteps that they'll encounter a lot of challenges as athletes during puberty. "What you need are knowledgeable coaches and parents who know how to support you during this time, to let you know it is normal, to celebrate you through development, who can zoom out on the big picture, because it is at this time that many girls give up," Lauren wrote. "You'll see girls react to a changing body in three ways: give up, ride it out, or fight against it. With 100 percent confidence, I can tell you the best choice is to ride it out. The best is yet to come."

THREE SIMPLE WAYS COACHES CAN TALK ABOUT PUBERTY

Every girl's experience through puberty and starting her period is different, but addressing what young athletes may experience as a result of this life stage will help them navigate it and, hopefully, keep them active throughout it.

- **Pool your resources.** Coaches who don't feel qualified to talk with girls about puberty and periods should ask for help; perhaps an athletic trainer or school nurse can start the dialogue with the team or ask the school administration to bring in a medical professional for a workshop. Invite older athletes to start a talking circle: the conversation begins by just prompting the athletes to talk about whatever is on their minds and gradually shifts as they become more comfortable with each other. Just creating opportunities for questions and information sharing can be enough to normalize the topic and make it less taboo.
- **Ask the team what they need.** Many girls and women we spoke to sing the praises of the coaches who were prepared with a supply of anything they might need. One male coach put together a bag that is always accessible with feminine hygiene products, pain

> relievers like Advil, and extra pairs of shorts. Anybody who needs
> something can just get it out of the bag—no questions asked.
> - **Remind them that periods are powerful.** Reinforce the message
>   that growing and menstruating are signs of strength and help young
>   athletes think of this stage as empowering. Periods are a sign of
>   health, and every athlete should want to be healthy.

MANAGING MENSTRUATION AND BREAST DEVELOPMENT

The culture on many sports teams doesn't make it easy for girls to ride it out, though. Meredith, the mother of two girls who ski, dance, and play volleyball, basketball, and soccer, whom we met in chapter 2, describes her teen daughter's soccer uniform, which includes white, formfitting shorts in a material so sheer that the players' underwear is visible. Every person who menstruates knows how problematic white bottoms can be—like the white skirts often required for tennis, for example. Mandating that girls, who may get their periods at inconsistent and inconvenient times, wear them can create such profound anxiety, it may well drive some players to simply quit. While sports can become a source of increased confidence, worrying about bleeding through a uniform surely takes away from self-esteem and concentration.

Meredith attends many soccer tournaments each season and notices when girls are missing from games or when they insist on wearing warm-up pants despite high temperatures, to avoid anyone seeing blood running down their legs. Then sometimes she wonders whether the obstacle is the uniforms or the portable toilets they must use, which lack a feminine hygiene disposal option inside, creating the embarrassment of using public garbage cans instead. Her own daughter has missed dance class when she has her period because she's had difficulty using tampons or menstrual cups, among the only options when you're required to wear a leotard to class. Young swimmers and water polo players can relate to that challenge as well. "I am disheartened by the lack of progress we have made for girls to feel uninhibited by their natural development," she says.

Periods are a natural bodily function that shouldn't come with stigmas attached, yet blood stains showing through a pair of shorts during a big game can become a mortifying ordeal.

Some professional women's sports are recognizing that small changes can help their players navigate the physical and emotional turbulence surrounding their periods. The Orlando Pride, for example, became the first team in the National Women's Soccer League to eliminate white shorts from its team uniform, replacing them with black bottoms that are less likely to show period leaks. The team announced the decision in February 2023, following the lead of Manchester City in October 2022, the first in the Women's Soccer League to make the call. Tennis players also advocated for the rule change at Wimbledon, which had traditionally mandated that all competitors dress in white. Now athletes are allowed to wear dark shorts underneath white shorts or skirts.

Haley Carter, the Pride's general manager and vice president of soccer operations, told *Women's Health*[4] that getting rid of unnecessary stressors during the time of a player's period is a no-brainer for improving outcomes. "But also, it normalizes conversations around periods, how menstruation can influence athlete performance, and how, culturally, we can navigate those conversations with our players."

Moves like the Pride's are also meant to serve as conversation starters for educating younger girls on the long-term risks involved in not getting their period, like cardiovascular disease, osteoporosis, and premature menopause. Cramps, bloating, mood fluctuations, bleeding, and fatigue are mostly normal and usually not an excuse to skip practices (unless a doctor advises otherwise); in fact, it's a moment to show them how exercise can help alleviate a lot of the less-desirable symptoms of menstruation. Endorphins, the hormones the body releases to relieve pain and reduce stress during activities, including exercise, can be a girl's best friend during that time of the month, even if running laps or lifting weights feel like the last things she wants to do. Sometimes we don't perform our best while we have our periods, but moving our bodies may help reduce a host of other issues, including premenstrual syndrome, the point at which many people feel anxious, depressed, tired, or just generally grumpy. Though it's still unclear, such symptoms may result from hormone changes or changes in brain chemicals; either way, they're real and affect athletic performance.

Attentive coaches also have a real impact in keeping girls active through the changes. Ally, for example, was an avid gymnast before she made the transition to acrobatics and tumbling. She was seventeen when she started her period, but her coaches openly and honestly educated their team about puberty and body changes—they even gave out kits with deodorant and period products. Ally never felt shy bringing up her cycle, which was lucky because so much of her life took place in the presence of her coaches. A changing body is especially difficult for gymnasts because it throws everything off. Girls have to adjust and reset runways, beams, bars, and balance. "It was scary to be launching off a vault, expecting it to feel how it felt countless times and now feels foreign," Ally says. "But our coaches were really supportive. It was never a taboo topic."

Girls also grapple with developing breasts that may hurt when they run, something they don't feel they can discuss with their male coaches. Sarah Lesko, who competed for Yale University track and field, was a family medicine physician and a track and cross-country coach for middle school girls. She's now the executive director of a nonprofit organization called Bras for Girls, which donates sports bras and breast development education booklets to girls in need, ages eight to eighteen, via sports teams, as well as school and community programs. The booklet that Bras for Girls has created details what girls can expect as their breasts grow and how everybody's development looks different. During a meeting with a potential partner, the male coach of a team said he agreed that Bras for Girls had a worthy mission but worried that the images of breasts in the educational material might make people uncomfortable. The whole point, of course, is to eliminate the stigma of talking about breasts and reduce one barrier for girls' participation in sports. A 2016 Portsmouth University survey of two thousand girls between the ages of eleven and seventeen found that 46 percent said their breasts affected their sports and exercise participation; 87 percent wanted to know more about breast development[5]; and one of the most common reasons they said that they didn't participate in sports was "I am embarrassed by excessive breast movement." Problems like this seem to have such obvious, easy solutions, thanks to organizations like Bras for Girls that are opening up the conversation.

THE POWER OF THE PERIOD

While increasing the number of women holding coaching positions at all levels of sport would ease the awkwardness of conversations surrounding issues like breast development, menstruation, and body image, male coaches should also learn how to address these issues, too. Men often feel ill-equipped to support girls in this way and, again, lack the educational opportunities to learn how to properly integrate women's health into their training philosophies. Coaches, regardless of gender, can become advocates for more comfortable uniforms, better bathroom facilities, and availability of period products for players.

Camille, a high school sophomore cross-country and track athlete, says her high school male coaches never had a conversation with the team about their periods. She knows that at least two girls hadn't menstruated for two years; one was running four times a day, and the other had been diagnosed with an eating disorder. When a female coach came on board, she asked everybody to track their cycles and talked about the health implications of amenorrhea. "People got lost on the JV team or didn't even know it's a bad thing they were losing their period," Camille says.

The bottom line? Female athletes are different from male athletes, biologically and physically. Shouldn't their training and conditioning regimens reflect those differences, instead of ignoring them? In 2019, the US Women's Soccer Team decided to learn more about how this could be achieved by tracking their menstrual cycles using an app called FitrWoman, which breaks the cycle down into four phases: menstruation (bleeding), follicular (six to ten days after bleeding), ovulation (when progesterone and estrogen increase), and luteal (premenstruation, when hormones decline).

Players learned what their bodies need most during each phase and how they're likely to feel, while their coaches helped them focus on proper rest, hydration, and nutrition throughout their cycles. In phase two, for example, women may feel more energized, and they are more likely to respond and adapt to high-intensity workouts during phases one and two. Fatigue often sets in during phase three and sleep can be disrupted, while appetite increases.

That year, the US Women's National Soccer Team won the World Cup. Not a bad endorsement for leveraging the power of the period (we can't say the effort resulted in the world title, of course, but it has encouraged more research and thoughtful consideration about how menstruation plays a role in athletic performance), or for the benefits of coaches learning more about how to adjust training based on individual needs. When coaches talk openly about periods and integrate female athlete needs into their programs, athletes become less fearful, more empowered, and develop more trust in their bodies.

Chapter Six

IDENTIFYING ANXIETY AND DEPRESSION

Girls and women are receiving diagnoses for these mental
health conditions at a higher rate than their male
counterparts. The signs and symptoms among
athletes may differ from others.

Cat, who began her collegiate swimming career at a Southeast Conference (SEC) program, knew she was struggling when she
returned to practice her sophomore year. Although she had already
competed at the international level as a high school athlete, the aftermath of that success had been tumultuous. As a teenager, she swam
under a club coach who had blamed her plateau in performance on her
weight, and she also suffered from overtraining syndrome (a mental
and physical breakdown that occurs when athletes push their bodies
beyond what they can adequately recover from in training), disordered
eating, and shoulder surgery. All of these factors contributed to her
declining mental health, which included depression.

When she went back to that SEC program, a new coach had taken
over and he was eager to cut swimmers from the roster. He fostered a
culture of fear every day, essentially setting expectations so high that it
was as if he was daring them to quit so he didn't have to do the dirty

work himself. Meanwhile, Cat had asked the team trainer for help in securing therapy. She waited several weeks, to no avail. Meanwhile, she pushed through difficult sets at practices, leaving her more depleted by the day. When a month had passed, she decided to find herself help outside of the university system and pay with her personal insurance but was told not to do so. Then she watched a higher-performing team-mate get access to a mental health professional within twenty-four hours of expressing her need. The knowledge that staff members had the power and responsibility to support her health and chose not to changed Cat's entire trajectory in the sport. "By the time I got in to see the therapist, I was already severely depressed. I was self-harming. I wasn't sleeping at all, either," Cat says.

Her healthcare provider prescribed medication, which Cat wasn't opposed to, but she immediately noticed unwanted side effects that made her question whether she was taking the right kind, in the correct dosage. She just felt "off," reporting nausea, fatigue, and aches, as well as worsening depression and increased suicidal ideation, she says. Despite her doubts and her body's reaction to the medication, the provider increased her dosage within four days, claiming it would help Cat compete at an upcoming meet that was important to the team. Cat didn't have the strength or energy to protest. "I just did what I was told," she says. "I didn't have any form of self-advocacy . . . asking to see a therapist was the best I could do. I never was the kind of person to question authority in any way."

Even under the circumstances, Cat still posted strong times at the meet. But her coaches remained unconvinced of her abilities and declined to add her to the travel roster, saying that her contributions were "unreliable." Slower teammates competed instead. After Cat's lowest point, a night in which she attempted suicide after reaching out to her trainer for support and receiving little help (as she remembers it, the trainer went so far as to say, "I'll see you at practice tomorrow"), she made plans to return home, swim for her club team, and regain her health.

Experiences like Cat's are replicated every day, in every sport and at every level, throughout the country, and so many athletes don't have the wherewithal to outright ask for help like she did. Female athletes are acutely aware that the stigma surrounding depression and anxiety still exists, and many fear that admitting they are coping with symptoms will lead to being labeled weak or lazy or worse, like getting cut from the team. But feeling sad or irritable, lacking energy, finding an inability to concentrate, and having a reduced appetite aren't great markers for athletic performance, either.

When an athlete sprains an ankle, she would likely receive immediate medical attention and a specific plan to get back to fitness as fast as possible. Yet the kind of care and attention athletes receive for physical ailments still does not extend to mental health conditions. Why? Stigmas and lack of education and resources for trainers and coaches are at least partly to blame; remember that the NCAA found in 2021 that only 50 percent of those competing for women's teams believed that their coaches took their mental health concerns seriously, and just 47 percent thought their athletic departments prioritized their mental health. Mental well-being may be evolving into a bigger part of the conversation within sports, but the talk is cheap unless it's backed by tangible resources and policies.

WHY WOMEN?

Women are almost twice as likely than men to have experienced depression and anxiety disorders at some point in their lives, according to the National Center for Health Statistics. Although it's more difficult to specify the prevalence of these conditions among athletes, the American College of Sports Medicine found in 2021 that 30 percent of female student-athletes competing at the collegiate level reported having anxiety—and that only 10 percent of all college athletes with known mental health conditions had sought care from a professional.

We know that people who exercise have better outcomes in managing depression and anxiety. Research has shown that even moderate activity like walking can enhance mood, releasing endorphins and other chemicals in the brain that make us feel better.[1] However, training and competing in sports can also trigger stress. High school and college athletes miss classes and schoolwork, the travel is disruptive to their routines and sleep patterns, and they often miss out on social activities outside of their sports, which can feel isolating—all while trying to maintain peak performance through many difficult transitions and milestones like moving away from home for the first time. They also face public scrutiny of their performances and behavior within their communities and beyond.

In a 2018 review of literature[2] concerning the psychology of female athletes, researchers found that risk factors for anxiety and depression include performance expectations, overtraining, sports-related injury, and involuntary career termination. This can be a vicious cycle. Athletes who have symptoms of anxiety also sustain injuries at a rate 1.9 times higher than those who don't, the research found. Anxiety and depression are also signs of overuse injuries and overtraining, as well as burnout.

According to the guidelines provided in the *Diagnostic and Statistical Manual of Mental Disorders*,[3] the standard for health care providers, anxiety is defined as an excessive feeling of fear or dread and uneasiness. It can cause a rapid heartbeat, restlessness, panic, sweat, and extreme nervousness or worry (this is more extreme than when somebody feels nervous about a test, for example). Depression is defined as a mood disorder that results in a persistent feeling of sadness and loss of interest in activities, decreased motivation, lack of energy, and loss of focus. People who are depressed often perceive the condition as permanent, like nothing they do will change how they feel. But the good news is that both anxiety and depression are highly treatable.

It is thought that hormone fluctuations and rapid body changes during puberty, premenstruation, postpartum, and during perimenopause and menopause could factor into higher rates of anxiety and depression in the general population of women. Women also live with many stresses that men don't, like unequal pay, meeting the demands of careers while remaining primary caregivers to children and aging parents, or coping with abuse or other safety concerns. But female athletes, as we have seen, often face additional stressors on top of these. We also know that athletes who experience chronic conditions that aren't due to acute circumstances (like a breakup or a death in the family, for example) may rely on exercise to mitigate their symptoms. The fact that these athletes will keep showing up for practice and appear high functioning makes it hard for parents, coaches, or even for the athlete herself to recognize that she's suffering from anxiety or depression— much less understand what factors contributed to the depression or anxiety to begin with.

AJ, a talented basketball player (who uses they/them pronouns), signed a letter of intent at seventeen years old with a NCAA Division I program, two years after they had been diagnosed with chronic major depressive disorder. At the time of their diagnosis, they were living with fatigue, feelings of worthlessness, self-harm, suicidal ideation, and a significantly restricted caloric intake. AJ now knows that they were experiencing the predictable results of an experience of sexual assault on the backdrop of intergenerational trauma, undiagnosed neurodivergence, and minority stress. After two years of therapy, they were making progress just as it was time to leave for college. But the combination of moving to another state, living in a dorm with a stranger, starting classes, and sustaining a long-distance romantic relationship was a lot to handle. "Predictably I really struggled during my freshman year," AJ says. "I found it incredibly difficult to manage the increased athletic and academic pressure and a matrix of new interpersonal relationships." Many of the symptoms AJ was living with became unmanageable. "I was constantly overwhelmed, often to the point of tears before, during, and after practices and games. Self-harming behaviors and suicidal ideation were prominent features of my daily life during that time."

An assistant coach offered AJ support and suggested that they consider medication—and AJ says that the antidepressants probably ended up saving their life multiple times. But that kind of suggestion, though made out of concern and care, shouldn't come from a coach, due to the inherent power imbalance, as well as the lack of qualifications to make that judgment. Coaches should extend curiosity and support and then connect athletes to the professionals who can explore the appropriate intervention. "I do think this encouragement would be more appropriate coming from someone who did not have control over things like my playing time or the status of my scholarship," AJ says.

AJ was encouraged to resume therapy but was connected with the clinical psychologist hired by the athletic department who specialized in sport performance, when what they really needed was somebody who specialized in treating post-traumatic stress. "The harsh reality is that the amount of staff allocated to student-athlete well-being is nowhere near sufficient," AJ says. "Folks fall through the cracks. Coaching and operational staff are not as equipped as they need to be in order to recognize and respond to signs that an athlete might be experiencing mental health distress. Nor is it fully acknowledged how incredibly common these experiences are for athletes."

AJ is correct. Many large athletic departments employ the equivalent of two full-time mental health professionals for every five hundred athletes. This allows these universities to say that team members have access to mental health care, even though they don't have enough staff to meet the demand.

Diagnosing depression and anxiety is nuanced, and not everybody presents the same symptoms. In our high school focus group, several athletes shared that they've been diagnosed with depression, one of whom says she's spent many days in bed, frequently missing school, which has impacted her participation in sports because she also misses practice time. Another young athlete describes feelings of self-loathing connected to her athletic performance—for every basket she misses, she tells herself that she's a terrible player and, in turn, a terrible person.

The hopelessness and loneliness lead her to thoughts of dying. Both athletes are experiencing depression, but each presents differently and their needs are different. That's exactly why these symptoms must be discussed with licensed professionals who understand the unique ways in which mental health conditions can manifest in athletes and understand the interventions needed.

MEDICATION AND ATHLETES

Many athletes wonder if their training and performance may suffer if they decide, with the help of a medical professional or prescriber, to take selective serotonin reuptake inhibitors (SSRIs) to treat anxiety or depression. Some worry that side effects will derail their efforts but also realize that medication may help alleviate the mental health symptoms they feel, which could also boost their motivation and drive.

The bottom line: taking SSRIs is often necessary and shouldn't come with shame or stigma. For those who are subject to drug testing in sports, it's important to be aware that SSRIs are not prohibited substances. Like any other supplement or prescription, antidepressant medication must be declared at the time of drug testing, but they are not banned, in or out of competition.

Still, athletes and coaches often hesitate. Amy, who competed on a cross-country team at a small college in the south, struggled with depression from her first year of eligibility. Her symptoms worsened, and she experienced panic attacks almost daily. After a suicide attempt in her sophomore year, she asked her doctor for a prescription, but when she told one of her coaches about it, the coach discouraged her from taking it until the season was over. "She said, 'You don't know how it's going to affect you. You might gain weight,'" Amy says. "I'm really glad I didn't listen to her."

It is true that these medications come with potential side effects. For example, antidepressant medication can increase suicidal thoughts for some people. It might be a temporary side effect that persists only while adjusting the medication, or it could be a sign that it is not the right medication for the individual. Either way, this is a conversation that must be had with a prescriber, which is why we, as clinicians, coordinate care with prescribers. First we ask the client if medication is an option they've considered or are curious about, then we share a referral list that we've created. Clients can then talk with a prescriber about potential side effects and determine the best path forward.

Amy went on a low dose of Fluoxetine and saw a difference within a few weeks. While some people feel a bit of a loss of their "edge" when taking an antidepressant, Amy felt lighter and freer—everything felt easier, including running. She just felt better. "Before, I had no energy or will to live. I just had complete loss of any emotion—I was void of feeling," Amy says. "And that's the most dangerous place to be because I was considering ending my life. The medication just kind of brought me back—I could feel things again and I felt alive again."

Every athlete is different, and for some people, getting the dosage adjusted to the right levels can take time and patience. Research on how it affects athletic performance is scattered and highly individual, but working with a psychiatrist, psychiatric nurse practitioner, or prescriber to find a medication that helps is vital. For many, like Amy, it can be lifesaving.

THE INJURY FACTOR

Often the presence of injury is strongly tied to bouts of depression and anxiety for female athletes. When a player gets hurt, she loses routine, physical activity, and the consistent interaction with teammates. She also often fears being out of shape or falling behind when she returns to sport, too—or if the injury is severe, she may also worry about whether a return to athletics will be possible at all.

Ann* was a Division II soccer player who attended a Christian-based institution, a school she found was the fit for her "academically, athletically, and spiritually." She was a talented player but had never anticipated

93

continuing soccer in college, so it was a pleasant surprise to find a place where she was excited to join the team. She was a starter her first year and her identity was quickly tied to soccer, which Ann couldn't have been more thrilled about. Then, in her sophomore year she began to feel pain in her hamstring during practice. "Being a college athlete, every practice is almost like a tryout for a starting spot or playing time," she says. "So I told myself to push through the pain because I didn't want to be seen as soft. When it was time for our first home game, I ended up straining my hamstring even more, and I tore it."

While she was sidelined, Ann feared she'd never be the same player she once was. She lost her confidence as well as her spot on the travel team. She watched her team grow and thrive without her, and even once she timidly returned to play, she was filled with anxiety. Still, by her junior year, Ann felt she needed soccer to be happy. "I felt only seen as an athlete. Even after I would have the best practice or game of my life, I would step back on the bus or get back to my dorm feeling so empty," she says. "I started to skip campus activities, my classes, and my meals just so I could stay confined in my room. My sociability, confidence, and overall energy felt drained."

Finally, Ann confided in her mother that she was struggling with depression. She sought help through her faith and counseling. She learned how to separate her performances on the field from how she felt about herself or her identity. "I still get episodes of feeling anxious or depressed, but now I know that it's OK."

The more they achieve in sports, the more athletes tie their identities to their athletic pursuits. It becomes hard to reconcile who they are when it's suddenly ripped away. Morgan Rodgers, for example, was a star lacrosse player for Duke University. During her senior year in high school, Morgan had been diagnosed with anxiety but received professional help that made her confident she'd succeed at college.

But just before Morgan's sophomore season, during practice, she went down hard with three tears in her ACL and MCL. It would take twelve months to return to the field, after surgery and relentless rehab.

Morgan's family believes that during that time, although she put on a happy and determined facade, on the inside she feared she was not living up to expectations and her self-esteem declined. Morgan felt isolated from her team, stressed by her relationships, and bogged down by anxiety and depression. She suffered alone and never let her loved ones know how much she was struggling. Morgan died by suicide in 2019, at the age of twenty-two.

Since her death, the Rodgers family and some of her friends started the nonprofit organization Morgan's Message, a national program that aims to eliminate the stigma surrounding mental health among the student-athlete community, normalize conversations, and equalize the treatment of physical and mental health in sports. The group has launched an ambassador program at colleges and youth sports organizations across the country where student-athlete volunteers are given much-needed resources and training to lead campus meetings and educational workshops about mental health.

CREATING SPACE

The instinct in sports is to push through, keep going, and eventually the hard work will lead to something good. But when we're concerned about anxiety or depression in an athlete, the solution is actually to slow down, pause, and allow the person to articulate what they are feeling and, if they can identify it, what they need. This can help uncover what's at the core of their symptoms. It might be a chronic condition, or it could stem from an acute circumstance. In talking with so many female athletes, we found that the athletic cultures themselves were creating circumstantial anxiety or depression, mostly in programs that are rigid and outcome-oriented. In these cases it was often the stress of the environment and the pressure to achieve results for coaches or parents, rather than an intrinsic desire to succeed, that was manifesting in mental health struggles.

It's not that athletes can't handle pressure or are unable to meet expectations in these systems, however. Some athletes work so hard and ultimately find no connection or fulfillment in this type of environment. The system itself is always going to demand more, no matter how much the athlete achieves. Sometimes the answer is to find a different setting. Olivia, for example, a swimmer at a large, prominent university in the southwest, had developed anxiety about her best event, the two-hundred-meter butterfly, as she was transitioning to college. She was one of the best in the country at the event and no doubt could become a big team contributor by competing in it, but the better she performed through the years, the more her panic grew. "I started having panic attacks whenever I had to swim it," she says. "I had put too much expectation on myself—I couldn't stop thinking about how nervous I was and how painful it would be."

Olivia opened up to her new coaches about her symptoms—and to her surprise, they met her with empathy, allowing her to choose whether to move to a new event or try the two-hundred-meter butterfly again. These coaches didn't do anything more than listen to and trust Olivia. They worked together to try to manage her anxiety, but when it didn't ease, they ultimately decided to switch events. "We wanted to let me have a fresh start and put more fun into the sport. We completely switched my NCAA lineup," Olivia says. "My college coaches are amazing. They're really big into having fun and not putting too much pressure on yourself."

Part of any successful intervention for athletes who are experiencing depression or anxiety is helping them reconnect to the joy they once felt for the sport and remember how to feel laughter and fun as a human, not just as an athlete. For some, like Olivia, it's switching up their focus, which can be rejuvenating. For others, it's giving them a chance to reconnect with their roots: to go home, sleep in their own bed, and visit their friends and families.

Loosening the reins and allowing that pause is therapeutic for young people experiencing high stress or sadness who may be feeling disconnected from the people and other activities that make them feel whole. The high school girls we spoke with, for example, described how their parents and coaches don't allow them to ski or go rock climbing because of the risk of injury. And while we agree that rules and policies during the competitive seasons are reasonable, we know that we can find ways to help athletes remain well-rounded and enjoy other activities. The high school girls also shared that coaches impose rules surrounding social media, threatening to bench anybody who uses it during the season. While social media certainly has its drawbacks for teen girls, it is also a primary way this demographic communicates with friends and plans social events (more on that coming in chapter 10). Giving athletes the space to learn how to manage their time, have a say in team policies, and find a sense of balance will help them avoid burnout.

Speaking of burnout, it's important for female athletes, as well as their parents and coaches, to understand and watch for the signs, which can mirror symptoms of depression—and sometimes an athlete can't tell the difference. Researchers Chris Stankovich and Timothy Neal have identified six main symptoms,[4] including diminished performance; physiological changes like elevated resting heart rate; cognitive changes (forgetfulness or decreased GPA); emotional issues like irritability, disinterest, or moodiness; behavioral changes (risk-taking, substance use); and immune system impairment leading to more colds or other illnesses. While burnout is a normal part of life (who hasn't experienced it at work or through parenting, for example?), for athletes, it has unique consequences because the ways in which most of us are able to cope with burnout—by taking breaks or switching our routines—are often unavailable.

Simone Manuel, who at the 2016 Rio Games became the first Black American woman to win an individual Olympic gold medal in swimming the hundred-meter freestyle, experienced all of those symptoms just months before the 2021 Olympic Trials. She was unable to qualify for the postponed Summer Games in her marquee event (she later qualified for the Games in the fifty-meter freestyle), disclosing afterward that she had been diagnosed with overtraining syndrome amid an otherwise difficult year. She had been training at Stanford University when the pandemic shut down facilities, leaving her to make do with access to a backyard pool. The escalating police violence against Black communities that summer drained her, too. She was compelled to speak up about racial injustice, including the killing of George Floyd.

When her performance at the Olympic Trials, which had been delayed by a year, didn't match expectations, Manuel spoke openly to the media[5] about her depression, overtraining, and all the variables that contributed to it. Just like anybody else, athletes are affected by the world around them, whether it's large societal issues or personal challenges. "Being a Black person in America played a part in it," Simone said. "It's not something I can ignore. It was just another factor that can influence you mentally in a draining way."

Her mental exhaustion and other symptoms also led Simone to isolate herself. "My mom would ask me questions on the phone and I would snap at her in ways I typically wouldn't," she said. "I had a hard time eating at times. I think the only way I got through it was talking to my loved ones and a sports psychologist."

Although complete rest was the only way for Simone to fully heal, she first had to prepare for the Tokyo Olympics. She came home with a bronze medal in the 4 x 100-meter freestyle relay and then, under doctor's orders, had to lay off all forms of exercise for several months. She spent time with her family, went to therapy, and allowed herself to grieve the experience she went through leading up to the 2021 Games. Then she found a new coach, Bob Bowman, who was Michael Phelps's longtime coach, and a training group that aligned with how she wanted to swim going forward, which included taking a slow progression to maintain her physical and mental health. She returned to the water in early 2023, telling SwimSwam[6] that she came back with a new "progress over perfection" perspective: "I get to swim and just kind of have fun doing it."

CHANGING THE ENVIRONMENT

Stories like Simone Manuel's and Morgan Rodgers's underscore the urgent need to make anxiety and depression screening a part of the overall wellness checks for athletes, especially when they're facing injuries and other events that pull them away from their sports. Unfortunately, psychological health isn't formally integrated into athlete care in most programs, and coaches aren't taught how to identify potential problems among their athletes, in contrast to the extensive physical exams required to compete.

Angelina Ramos, assistant track and field coach at Ball State University and former coach at the University of Nevada, Las Vegas, has taken to creating opportunities to check in with her runners at times they aren't focused on training, like walking to classes or study halls with them, especially when she senses they may need to talk. She doesn't hesitate to help them access mental health resources and tries to remain connected to those who have expressed they are struggling. But sustaining these important conversations takes a lot of time. Being the only female coach on staff adds another element of pressure to remain available, even when she's traveling or spending time with her own family. So much of the load that coaches carry is invisible and immeasurable.

Like Angelina, most coaches feel an overwhelming sense of commitment to their athletes, but they also don't have the expertise to treat anxiety or depression. While most athletic departments have a clear protocol and policy when somebody is injured, it is less clear what a coach is supposed to do about a mental health concern, although they are de facto mental health first responders as the adult who most often interacts with these young people and observes their daily behavior.

If a runner has a sprained ankle, the trainer, massage therapist, physical therapist, and coach would take a team approach to treatment and recovery. The coach would receive updates on how it's feeling and when the medical team thought it would clear the athlete to return to practice. Angelina would like to see a similar protocol for mental health, allowing the same kind of updates each week that include input from the student-athlete's academic advisor, therapist, dietician, and other people on the support team who could share patterns and progress (without violating HIPAA, obviously). It'd be a way to spot behavioral changes earlier and address early indicators of mental health needs.

"A counselor's or therapist's ability to help is sometimes limited by an athlete's self-awareness. If they can't see it and I, as a coach, can't communicate it to them, we are not supporting the athlete and it is unlikely services will be as effective," Angelina says. "I don't need to know all the details about somebody's therapy session, but coaches would like to hear recommendations of things to watch or look for. A heads up, like 'be kind, or be lenient on this today,' for example."

One way to help athletes open doors of communication is preseason agreements. While medical professionals are bound by law to keep patient information confidential, athletes may want to allow members of their support team to communicate about their health (mental and physical) and well-being. This removes coaches from taking on roles they shouldn't—like, therapist, for example. Preseason mental health evaluations or surveys could also serve as baseline data to refer to when needed later in the year—similar to the baseline concussion evaluations that athletes receive.

We know that the current piecemeal approach within sports is mostly reactionary to symptoms of anxiety and depression rather than preventative. We need to shift from treating these conditions to changing the systems that perpetuate them. Athletics is a perfect place to construct the framework for early intervention. Symptoms of anxiety and depression are normal, but sometimes those symptoms become intense and long-lasting. It's crucial that both athletes and coaches feel like they have the knowledge and resources to recognize, monitor, and take appropriate steps to address the symptoms that emerge.

Chapter Seven

IDENTIFYING MISTREATMENT AND ABUSE

Verbal, emotional, physical, and sexual abuse
within sports results in life-long trauma.

Few of us will ever forget watching the more than one hundred gymnasts stand up in court in 2018, one by one, and confront their abuser, Larry Nassar. It was a pivotal and difficult moment in the history of women's sports, to recognize the tragedy, to witness their anger, and to discover how every system, at every level, had failed to protect the safety and well-being of some of the country's most revered athletes.

Over four days in the Lansing, Michigan, courtroom, the judge allowed 156 girls and women to describe the decades of sexual assault they endured while under the doctor's "care." They described how Nassar's abuse led to lifelong anxiety, depression, suicidal thoughts, family breakdowns, and more. Some could remember assaults beginning when they were as young as six years old. By the end of their testimony, Nassar was sentenced to up to 175 years in prison for criminal sexual conduct. But for the gymnasts, the fight for justice is not over. They have remained stalwart, pushing for more accountability and advocating at the highest levels for reform. Simone Biles, seven-time Olympic medalist, was one of the athletes who spoke before members of Congress in

2021, demanding that officials take responsibility for athlete welfare. "I don't want another young gymnast, Olympic athlete, or any individual to experience the horror that I and hundreds of others have endured—before, during, and continuing to this day in the wake of the Larry Nassar abuse. To be clear, I blame Larry Nassar, and I also blame an entire system that enabled and perpetrated his abuse," Simone said to the Senate Judiciary Committee.[1]

Evidence presented at trial revealed that officials at USA Gymnastics (the sport's governing organization), the US Olympic and Paralympic Committee, Michigan State University (where Nassar was employed), and even the FBI had failed to act on reports from athletes and parents, declined to call authorities or pursue investigations, and perpetuated a culture of secrecy and abuse for decades. Authority figures, including club-level coaches, failed to take action for nearly twenty-five years, until the *Indianapolis Star*[2] published an investigation in 2016 with the help of a few athletes who were willing to tell their stories when nobody else would. By doing so, they put a perpetrator in prison and shined a national spotlight on the ugly underbelly of Olympic sports. Their example also gave an untold number of other female athletes permission to speak out about the trauma they, too, have endured.

What we've learned since then—or perhaps recognized more publicly—about the degree to which abuse is pervasive in girls' and women's sports has shocked the nation. But why? Sports leagues, an arena created for men and by men, have always been a place where the fear of punishment, whether it's physical (running laps if you're late for practice) or verbal (lots of yelling and screaming)—is ingrained. Such tactics make players "tough," they say, a term of praise and endearment for those involved in sports. Athletes who experience bullying, hazing, or sexual harassment, for example, often don't report it because they fear for their playing time and their athletic careers, worry about rejection from teammates, or are concerned that nobody will believe them—and they simply don't know who to tell, either. What if saying something just makes a player appear weak? Like she just can't handle it?

Emotional and verbal mistreatment are so normalized that many players don't recognize it as abuse until after they stop playing and gain perspective. Girls and women often find themselves in controlling environments, answering to older men (due to their continued dominance in sport leadership positions), without any power in these relationships, and if that mistreatment is coming from a coach, the power imbalance is often too much to overcome. Combine all that with the fact that, until the past few years raised awareness about the kinds of abuse that athletes experience, little training or education has been mandated to help athletes, parents, coaches, and officials identify or prevent abuse, and it's easy to see how the system itself has enabled abuse to occur.

In one effort to try to address the issues, the US Center for SafeSport was founded in 2017 as a nonprofit organization, designated by the US Congress to respond to reports of sexual misconduct within US Olympic and Paralympic sports. Under the Protecting Young Victims from Sexual Abuse and Safe Sport Authorization Act, its mandate is to develop policies to prevent emotional, physical, and sexual abuse of athletes of all ages participating in Olympic sports at every level, from youth to elite (it covers eleven million athletes, coaches, and other officials, in fifty sports, it says, but among its shortcomings is that it has no jurisdiction over the NCAA or other collegiate-level associations, for example). Funding for the center comes from the US Olympic and Paralympic Committee, the Department of Justice, foundations, and donors. Officials, coaches, and volunteers are often required to take SafeSport certification training, and the center also keeps an online public database of those serving suspensions or who are under investigation.

As more people understand the center's existence and purpose, more investigations are piling up. In 2021, the center received 3,708 reports of abuse and misconduct, which was 60 percent more than in 2020.[3] One criticism of the efforts has been that the investigations and resolutions have taken too long and that the center is overwhelmed (and underfunded), though officials at the center say that the backlog of investigations has diminished. It investigated 18 percent more cases in

2021 than in 2020. Others have called the center "a paper tiger" that lacks transparency and hasn't earned the trust of the population it's supposed to serve. "If you're SafeSport, and you're funded by the organization you're investigating, they're likely not going to do the right thing,"[4] said Aly Raisman, two-time Olympic gymnast, during her testimony before the Senate Judiciary Committee in 2022.

It's clear that athletes have needed somewhere to turn to (aside from law enforcement, where all reports should start for anybody who's been physically or sexually assaulted—though the criminal justice system also suffers a backlog of processing rape kits). According to its own 2021 survey of four thousand adult athletes in more than fifty sports, the center found that 93 percent of athletes who experienced sexual harassment or unwanted sexual contact did not report it.[5] About 80 percent indicated they have experienced at least one of eighteen indicators of psychological harm (examples include stalking, verbal attacks like body-shaming or name-calling, or physical acts like throwing equipment or punching walls) or neglect (denying attention or support or excluding somebody intentionally for no productive reason)—and athletes with disability, women, and gender-nonconforming people experienced higher rates compared with men. About 9 percent of respondents said they had experienced inappropriate sexual contact during their sports involvement, mostly by coaches, trainers, administrators, or peer athletes. Black athletes and bisexual athletes experienced nearly double the rates of inappropriate sexual contact.

WHAT IS ATHLETE-CENTERED COACHING?

In the wake of the Nassar abuse scandal, USA Gymnastics[6] has provided resources regarding abuse and what parents and athletes should look out for within their clubs, which apply to all sports. Among the guidance is how to recognize quality coaching and what sets it apart from emotionally abusive situations. Here's what kind of culture you want to see:

- Doesn't use personal attacks, belittling, or degradation to "motivate"
- Focuses on sport-specific corrections, avoiding critiques about personality or appearance, for example
- Athletes look forward to practice even when it's difficult
- Coaches don't raise their voices in a demeaning manner to drive training or performance
- Relationships are built on mutual respect and coaches seek to solve problems when questions arise
- Coaches admit their mistakes to athletes
- Health and welfare are the first priority

Other attributes that coaches should have:

- Encourages athletes to have outside interests and respects that each player deserves a personal life
- Cultivates a trust-based relationship and values caregivers as a stakeholder in the athlete's process
- Allows the athlete freedom to make choices about participation and well-being

RECOGNIZING ABUSE

Researchers have established that sports encourage, and in some cases demand, obedience from participants, which teaches them from a young age to suppress emotions, including fear, anxiety, or anger associated with mistreatment or abusive behavior by coaches. That makes it difficult for caregivers to identify any problems their young athletes may encounter, but we know that at least 50 percent of women will experience some form of trauma in their lives, according to the National Alliance of Mental Illness.[7] It is four times as high for people who are gender diverse, transgender, and nonbinary.[8] It's beneficial to discuss with athletes at age-appropriate levels throughout their athletic careers about abuse and how to identify adults or officials they can always talk to if something feels bad or wrong.

Trauma itself is an all-encompassing term that includes all kinds of abuse and the aftermath (we will dive deeper into processing post-career trauma in chapter 12). Natalie Gutiérrez, a therapist who works with Black, Indigenous, and people of color who are survivors of complex trauma, describes trauma as "the imprint of chronic, toxic stress in our minds and bodies. It's the powerlessness we feel when we cannot over-come something, or someone, causing us immense pain. Trauma robs us of our self-love and completely changes our sense of safety in the world."[9] Judith Herman, a renowned psychiatrist and expert on trau-matic stress, called trauma "an affiliation of the powerless." "Traumatic events overwhelm the ordinary systems of care that give people a sense of control, connection, and meaning," Herman says. "They confront human beings with the extremities of helplessness and terror, and evoke the responses of catastrophe."[10]

It's important to think about trauma as a wide range of experiences. Sometimes we assume it must be a major event to be considered trau-matic. Clinically, we like to think about incidents of significant or vast proportions (sexual assault, gun violence, death of a parent, for exam-ple) as "Big T" trauma. Instances that are distressing but don't fit that "Big T" category (like job loss or a friend breakup) are classified as "lit-tle t" trauma. We should hold space for the many different forms of traumas that can occur because what isn't traumatic for us may be for someone else. Widening the definition allows for a multitude of experi-ences and for the multitude of reactions that people have to those expe-riences. From where we sit, it isn't useful to decide somebody else's type of trauma.

Trauma survivors have experienced severe stress and have overactive stress responses, which is why something that most members of a team might see as a minor incident may cause a teammate who has experi-enced abuse to react with aggression or, alternatively, may cause that person to become overwhelmed or completely shut down. Sometimes trauma presents psychosomatically through symptoms like headaches or stomach pain. Experts have categorized the trauma response in four ways: fight (sudden anger or aggression), flight (shutting down emotionally, isolating, not communicating), freeze (showing no reaction or emotion), or fawn (avoiding conflicts, people-pleasing). It's helpful to remember what researchers and practitioners have long said: we all react to trauma differently. Within athletic systems, turning toward athletes with curiosity is critical. We don't know what's going on, and the athlete isn't under any obligation to tell anybody. But keeping in mind that people experience trauma in many ways and suspending assumptions about why an athlete is behaving a particular way goes a long way toward helping them.

Emily, the swimmer who started her NCAA career at an SEC D-I program with a toxic, fear-based culture, recalls how "terrified" she was during those years. "I tried to be perfect in everything that I did to avoid getting yelled at," she says. "I was told by a senior that I was a 'waste of f**king lane space.' There were so many other instances of small traumas that occurred; I was completely miserable, but transferring felt like it would be a failure."

TYPES OF ABUSE IN SPORTS:

Physical. Aggressive or violent behavior that results in bodily injury, like punching, kicking, biting, choking, shaking, throwing equipment at an athlete, hazing, shoving, denying hydration or nutrition, or punishing athletes through excessive exercise. It can also include ignoring an athlete's injury or forcing somebody to train or compete while injured.

Emotional (also called psychological abuse). Experts do not have a universal definition yet for emotional abuse, but it is a pattern of behavior that deliberately and repeatedly subjects another to acts that are detrimental to overall mental well-being. It can include

> verbal abuse, intimidation, humiliation, degradation, harassment, excessive control, and isolation. In sports, it can show up as a coach refusing, as a form of punishment, to give directions or feedback to an athlete, body-shaming or promoting disordered eating, scapegoating, or belittling.
>
> **Verbal.** Extremely critical, threatening, or insulting words delivered in oral or written form, intended to demean, belittle, or frighten somebody, as defined by the American Psychological Association. It might look like an athlete is being bullied, either by another athlete or a coach.
>
> **Sexual.** Violation or exploitation by sexual means. It includes any sexual contact between an adult and a child but can occur in any relationship of trust—eight out of ten sexual assaults are perpetrated by somebody known to the survivor. An athlete who has been sexually abused may have experienced a request of a sexual act, indecent exposure or exposure to pornographic materials, fondling, penetration, or rape.

It may take many years for an athlete suffering from the effects of trauma to identify exactly what they experienced. Lynn Jennings, now in her sixties and retired as an Olympic bronze medalist and one of the most accomplished women's long-distance runners in US history, for example, was sexually abused beginning at age fifteen by her coach, John Babington, and didn't investigate what happened until she was well into her fifties. In a report by the *Boston Globe* in 2023,[11] Lynn revealed that Babington had sexually assaulted her multiple times, including at the Olympic Trials in a University of Oregon dorm room. But at age seventeen, she was running some of the best times in the country and her star was rising, so she buried it. "I knew that if I said anything, it would have been taken away from me, the thing that I loved," Lynn told the *Globe*, in the February 2023 article. "I became a whiz at compartmentalizing."

What Lynn didn't realize until much later was that Babington had gone on to sexually assault other female athletes, including in 1996 while he was a coach at Wellesley College. He was fifty-one years old, the Wellesley athlete was nineteen, and although the runner and her parents reported the assault to the college officials, Babington was not fired, but placed on an unpaid leave for just one cross-country season. He remained in the position until he retired in 2013. For its part, Wellesley issued a lengthy statement[12] after the February 2023 *Globe* story was published, reiterating its policies and said, in part, "The fact that this happened at Wellesley, a college dedicated to the education and advancement of women, speaks to the ubiquity of this problem."

The statutes of limitations had expired on all of Babington's offenses, which allowed him a full coaching career. He is now permanently banned by the US Center for SafeSport, thanks to Lynn's investigative work tracking down other survivors and corroborating her own story. "I am unburdened now in ways I have never been since I was fifteen years old. Telling what happened has freed me," Lynn told the *Globe*.

So many coaches remain well-intentioned, caring role models who show compassion and dedication to the well-being of their athletes and provide a safe place for those athletes to learn and grow. Certainly, the entire coaching profession should not be demonized. And yet, we also have to recognize the ways in which power imbalances and sport systems are allowing harmful behavior to continue. We place trust in the organizations and people who help our children succeed, and desired results like championship titles and scholarships can reinforce our belief in the people who are guiding our kids' athletic careers. When everything is on the line—the opportunity to make the varsity team, go to college, or even win an Olympic medal—traumatized athletes are not in a position to seek help; and the system isn't set up to offer it without consequence. The result is that girls and women often find themselves in controlling environments without any power in these relationships.

The US Women's Soccer League investigation, triggered by accusations first uncovered by the *Washington Post*[13] and *The Athletic*,[14] provides a sobering example. Although several were implicated, the investigation focused on three coaches in particular: former Chicago Red Stars coach Rory Dames; Christy Holly, former Racing Louisville FC coach; and Paul Riley, former coach of the North Carolina Courage. According to the investigation, Holly invited a player to his home to watch game film but instead showed pornography and masturbated in front of her. Another time, he groped the player's genitals and breasts each time he saw her make a mistake on the film. Holly was also accused of verbal abuse and creating a "toxic team environment" due to a relationship with a player. Riley was accused of using his position to coerce three players into sexual relationships and of being verbally abusive during his time coaching the Portland Thorns. Dames, who also coached youth teams, was alleged to have spoken to young players about their sex lives, screamed at them, belittled them, and "crossed the line to sexual relationships," according to the investigators' report. We know that in these circumstances, the athlete finds herself wrestling with her own shock about what's happening, often freezing and fearful because the perpetrator is in such a position of power over her safety and career—her playing time, salary, and more.

As we've mentioned, currently, to coach or get involved in leading a sport, all one typically needs is a clear criminal background check and perhaps a SafeSport certification, which anyone can get by taking an easy online class. This is how the Larry Nassars and John Babingtons continue to bounce from one program to another; it's easy to gain access and avoid getting caught, and so few people are trained to identify abuse or abusers. Perpetrators are often masters at manipulating their victims and even those who are close to their victims (family members, close friends, and more) to win their trust. They often isolate their victims from their loved ones, making up excuses and suggesting that the athlete needs to focus or rest; they share secrets with their victim that make it seem like they have a special relationship; and they start by hugging or other "harmless" touching and escalate from there as boundaries break down and the athlete becomes desensitized to such contact.

It should go without saying that when sexual abuse occurs, it's disorienting and violating, which is why it may take years or decades for an athlete to acknowledge it or talk about it. At the time, an assault makes no sense to the survivor, and often, the survivor doesn't think anybody will believe it happened, especially as this is so often the case when the perpetrator enjoys a reputation as a successful, trustworthy person. It becomes easy for an entire system to forsake the safety of the athletes for the winning record of a charismatic, likable, winning coach.

TOUGH COACHING OR EMOTIONAL ABUSE?

Olivia, the swimmer at a prestigious southwestern NCAA program, plainly calls her high school club experience "traumatic." Her coach used fear-based strategies to get results, threatening the team with harder sets, restarting sets so practices would run longer, and yelling at them from the deck whenever he spotted something he didn't like. "If you didn't swim fast, there was a high chance that he called you stupid, an idiot, and other degrading names," Olivia says.

She specifically recalls that one day after practice, the coach gave every girl a fifteen-pound weight to hold over their heads and told them that was how much weight they each needed to lose. The following day, one girl hid in the locker room out of fear. The coach sent his wife in to get her so he could reinforce his demands from the previous practice. "I remember not being able to intervene and stop it, just watching [my teammate] sob in front of everyone," Olivia says. "At swim meets, he would yell in our faces about how shitty we swam and cuss us out on the pool deck."

For Cat, the swimmer who competed for an NCAA Southeast Conference program, anxiety, depression, self-harm, and suicidal ideation escalated as she advanced through her sport and endured various forms of abuse. She distinctly recalls her club coach calling the girls "fat burritos" during practices. When she qualified for the world championships, it was hard to refute his mistreatment because she was producing high-caliber results. But when she developed a serious shoulder injury, he told her it was "all because you gained weight," and demanded she train for six hours a day. She was overtraining and was expected to hit the same time intervals as her male teammate who had also made the world team. "I fully bought into my coach's mind games," Cat says.

It seems that emotional abuse goes hand-in-hand with the masculine culture of sports, in some ways. And it isn't only perpetuated by male coaches, either. Teri McKeever, the former swim coach at the University of California, Berkeley for twenty-nine years, was fired in 2022, after an eight-month investigation that resulted in a five-hundred-page report detailing years of bullying, abuse, discrimination toward swimmers with disabilities, and racist behavior toward Black athletes. In response, Teri planned to file a civil lawsuit against the university based on gender discrimination. In December 2023, the US Center for Safe-Sport issued Teri a coaching suspension for emotional misconduct.

"Because she's a female she's supposed to respond in a nurturing way. She's supposed to be more attentive to the athletes, more caring of the feelings of athletes," her attorney told the OC Register.[15] "And when Teri McKeever and other females do not respond in that expected way the athletes assume that she's being critical of them in a very specific way." We would counter that all coaches should avoid verbally (and of course physically) abusing athletes and that they all hold *themselves* to the same standards, no matter their gender identity.

So, what's considered emotional abuse? It's any behavior meant to stoke fear, to belittle, or to humiliate, and it includes taking advantage of an imbalance of power. It can manifest in yelling or screaming, inconsistent affect (hot and cold) toward the players, name-calling, inappropriate jokes at an athlete's expense, gaslighting, attempts to isolate a player from her teammates, and ongoing attacks on an athlete's appearance, character, or athletic performance. The abuser can usually manipulate parents or other observers into thinking they are just demanding discipline from the players, but chances are, if you find yourself "walking on eggshells" constantly, the behavior constitutes emotional abuse.

Amy was about to embark on a promising four years as a distance runner for a southern Christian college. She arrived on campus inexperienced and admittedly a bit naive. Within the first few months of classes and practices, a fellow track athlete at a neighboring university asked her to hang out at his apartment. What she thought was an innocent night watching a movie ended in sexual assault, she says. Amy was traumatized and ashamed. It didn't take long until she started experiencing symptoms of depression. Her performance declined along with her mental health. Meanwhile, teammates informed her that their coach was gossiping with them, spreading rumors that Amy was "sleeping around," and isolated her from the group.

She started having panic attacks before races, terrified of the consequences if she didn't run well. In one instance, she began crying at a meet and an assistant coach told her to stop; crying just wasn't allowed. Finally, her roommate, one of the few people Amy had confided in, encouraged her to tell her coach that she had been sexually assaulted and was suffering in the aftermath. So Amy spoke with her coach. She remembers him saying, "boys will be boys" and that he had also "had his fun" as a college student. She needed to move on—and perform better for the team, he told her. It was a life-altering moment for Amy. "That one conversation could have changed everything for me, if I had been shown absolutely any care or been given any real help," she says. "It wasn't that he didn't believe me, it was just that he didn't care. When an athlete tells you something like that, coaches should have the resources or the education for how to approach that kind of conversation." Instead, Amy became further ostracized and her privacy breached.

"At a team retreat that fall, we had a big confrontational meeting and everyone was given an opportunity to tell me how negative I was and how I was faking feeling sick and hurt," Amy says. "I was put on the spot by my coach to share the reason I wasn't OK, which was incredibly violating." Amy attempted suicide, though a friend intervened and stayed with her for several hours (in retrospect, Amy believes she should have sought immediate medical attention, but she saw her doctor soon after, who prescribed antidepressant medication). She went back to practice the next day and continued to compete through injuries, illnesses, and continued emotional abuse. When she was given the choice to retain her scholarship and stay home during the COVID-19 year, which was her last, she took it. Despite reports to the college officials, meeting with a Title IX officer (under Title IX, federally funded colleges and universities must respond to reported sexual harassment and sexual violence), and filing a SafeSport report, the coach remained in his position without any consequences. "I see new girls sign up to run for him and wonder who will be his next target," Amy says. "I feel helpless because no one with the power to protect them has done anything."

Racism, sexism, and other forms of discrimination also constitute abuse. The report from the US Women's Soccer League investigation also detailed the league's "long-standing failure to adequately address racism and racially insensitive remarks," highlighting the lack of diversity in the sport and the racism that young Black girls experience from parents and teammates. Dames, in particular, was noted for making "sexist and racist remarks to players and retaliated against . . . players when they spoke out." Among the report's recommendations was that teams be required to vet coaches and suspend licenses of those who commit misconduct; that teams should each designate someone within their organizations who is responsible for player safety; and teams should disclose misconduct to the league and US Women's Soccer so that coaches are no longer able to move from one team to the next.

The examples are endless. Every girl and woman we talked with—hundreds of them—had an example of bullying, hazing, body-shaming, and more. Few were ever able to find help or successfully report an abuser. Verbal and emotional abuse is often still written off as "tough coaching," but that's an outdated and, frankly, lazy way of leading athletes. And long-term, it doesn't produce results, either.

DEFINING TYPES OF ABUSE AND WHAT TO DO IF YOU SUSPECT IT

Abuse shows up in a variety of ways—some are unique to the sports environment while others are not. Within sports, the abuser can be a coach, trainer, support staff, peer athlete, or parent. Different types of abuse can happen simultaneously and, of course, people of all genders can be victims just as people of all genders can be abusers.

If you suspect child abuse: If you suspect a child is being abused or neglected, first make sure to create a safe space where she can talk and be reassured that she is believed and what has happened is not her fault. Then look up the department in your state that receives reports of child abuse (note that you only have to suspect that an incident has occurred—you do not have to be certain). If it's an emergency situation, call 911. You can also call Childhelp USA (800-4-A-CHILD) or your local child protective services agency. After the initial reports are made to law enforcement, also contact the US Center for SafeSport to investigate.

If you suspect abuse of an adult athlete: Admittedly, this situation is tricky. Experts suggest finding a safe time and place to talk to somebody (away from practice or practice facilities) who you feel is in an abusive situation. Ask if you can offer support and recognize that although the athlete may reject it, they now know that you are available, should she change her mind at any time. Begin documenting any examples or signs of abuse that you observe with dates and as many details as you can, in case the athlete decides to report it to authorities. If you are a mandatory SafeSport reporter, contact the US Center for SafeSport and file a report.

CULTURES OF ABUSE

Though they dictate the culture of a team and can stoke mistreatment among their athletes, it's not just coaches who are perpetrating the abuse. Audrey*, for example, was on a university acrobatics and tumbling team, hoping to find balance between athletics, academics, and her social life at a large Division I school. She connected with a fellow athlete on Instagram—a highly recruited five-star football player—and developed a crush. They started casually dating. One night while at his apartment, they were having consensual sex, but she discovered that he was secretly filming them. Audrey confronted him, but he didn't feel like it was a big deal and refused to delete the recording. He laughed while Audrey felt violated and powerless. "In the moment I was scared because I clearly couldn't trust this man and was worried what could happen. Could he get violent? Was he going to feel bad? What was he going to do next? All these things were going through my head."

Like many other women in similar circumstances, Audrey believed that she had no recourse. He was the most admired athlete on campus. It was her word against his. Nobody ever talked about what to do if something happened to make you feel unsafe, especially at the hands of another athlete. "I also knew that he was a high-profile athlete, and would anyone believe me over him? So I kept it all in and never told anyone," Audrey says. "Unfortunately, we crossed paths many times after because we were both athletes . . . I would walk past with my head down and he would look away."

Erika, another standout D-I swimmer, also encountered plenty of turmoil in the form of bullying and belittling from other people in her program, she says. Still, it was hard to say no to a full-ride scholarship, so Erika tried to roll with it. When she moved into her room and met her new roommate, she immediately felt uncomfortable, beyond the usual awkward transition period when you're living with a stranger. The roommate became highly critical of Erika, down to her wardrobe. The team put the first-year recruits through an extensive hazing process, which entailed a lot of drinking, dancing in front of the men's team while the men threw cups of alcohol and trash at them, and other demeaning activities. And within those first few weeks she discovered that the full-ride she was promised was actually $20,000 short of a full-ride, per year. This was a considerable amount of money she didn't think her family could cover.

When her parents came for a short visit, Erika jumped into the back seat of the car and told them to take her home. Even though she didn't want to let them down, she knew the environment was unsafe. While Erika's dad wanted her to see her commitment through, her mom recognized that something was wrong. They decided that breaking a contract and taking a year of ineligibility was best. But when Erika came back to campus to tie up loose ends, her coach requested a meeting. When she arrived, the entire team was in the room, and he demanded she address each woman about why she was leaving. "It reinforced my decision," Erika says. A year later, the coach was fired for having sexual relations with his athletes. Then he was hired by another university. And the cycle continues.

As therapists, we hear repeatedly how survivors of abuse and violence don't tell anyone because they have heard that the likelihood of justice is small after they've been violated. It's the responsibility of the leadership, from league presidents and university presidents to coaches and athletic directors, to create safe and respectful environments where abuse of any kind is not tolerated. And we know that the culture of silence expands way beyond athletics—we also believe that law enforcement and the justice system have a lot of work to do in ensuring the safety of all.

Chapter Eight

COPING WITH BODY IMAGE AND EATING DISORDERS

Athletes are especially at risk.

Cross-country skier Jessie Diggins made history at the 2022 Beijing Winter Olympics as the first American woman to medal in the 1.5-kilometer freestyle sprint, taking home the bronze to sit alongside the gold she won in 2018 in the freestyle team sprint, with Kikkan Randall. The media coverage of this significant achievement included this analysis from the *New York Times*[1]: "In a sport that has so many women with massive shoulders and thighs, Diggins looks like a sprite in her racing suit, and it's not clear exactly where she gets her power."

The backlash was swift, from all corners of women's sports, and called on sports writers and broadcasters to cease commenting on the bodies and physiques of athletes and focus instead on the training and racing strategies that have led these women to podium finishes. Some asked if journalists receive any mental health education about how their word choices can be harmful, especially for young girls who are watching from afar, wondering what it might take to reach their own athletic goals—or whether they'd even want to pursue such dreams if it meant their bodies might be compared, critiqued, and criticized so publicly in the process. And, as most people who follow cross-country skiing know, Jessie has been vocal about her struggle with bulimia during her late teens. At every race, she dons the logo of the Emily Program, where she received treatment for her eating disorder, on her headband, and became an outspoken advocate for eating disorder awareness and recovery after revealing her story in 2018.

Instead of a celebratory Instagram post[2] after her momentous performance, Jessie chose to address what she deemed her "most important takeaway" from the 2022 Olympics, the one she says she would have needed to hear when she was a teen. "I was only able to get to those start lines because I am healthy, happy, and have a loving and supportive team around me. Listening to my body and taking good care of it isn't something I've always done, but getting help for my eating disorder and learning to accept my strengths instead of always trying to be 'perfect' is why I'm still racing today." Jessie went on to explain why the remarks in the *Times*, contrasting the bodies of female athletes competing in her event, were damaging—and clarifying what she believes has led to success on the world stage: "being a great teammate, mental strength, competing clean, training with purpose and racing with guts."

As a talented and fiercely competitive skier and gifted student in high school, Jessie has described herself as a classic perfectionist, always striving for 100 percent, all the time. It spurred chronic stress at a young age, when her body was naturally going through a lot of growth and change, which she numbed with her eating disorder. It gave her the sense that she was in control of something, when everything else felt out of control, Jessie wrote in her 2018 blog.[3] "You can't give someone an eating disorder. You don't get one from looking at photos of skinny, ripped athletes. Can it be a trigger for some people? Absolutely," she wrote.

What Jessie describes is the complexity of eating disorders, which can stem from genetics, but can also be triggered by the environment. Some people are more susceptible than others because of innate personality traits, but that doesn't mean a person will necessarily develop one. It depends on many individual factors.

As mentioned, one factor is the environment, which includes coaches or caregivers who monitor food consumption, fixate on weight and body composition, and perpetuate team cultures of eating disorders, as well as media attention on appearance, society's obsession with diet culture, and the ongoing assumption that the "ideal" body—what we've learned to believe is the norm—is lean and white.

DIAGNOSING EATING DISORDERS

It's been difficult to nail down exact figures, but research consistently estimates that up to 45 percent of female athletes experience eating disorders or disordered eating at some point in their lives.[4] Another study of Division I NCAA athletes showed that one-third of women in sports reported attitudes and symptoms that placed them at risk for anorexia nervosa.[5] The National Association of Anorexia Nervosa and Associated Disorders (ANAD) says that almost twenty-nine million Americans will have an eating disorder in their lifetime.[6] And, as the pandemic took hold in 2020, hospitalizations for eating disorders spiked to all-time highs among teen girls.

These are mental and physical illnesses that affect people, regardless of gender, age, ethnicity, or sexual orientation. What spurs them? Expert opinions are varied, but it is different for everybody. They are caused by a combination of factors including biological (having a close relative with an eating disorder or mental health condition; a history of dieting or weight control), psychological (perfectionism, body image dissatisfaction, anxiety disorder, or "behavioral inflexibility," which is a fancy way of saying "devout rule follower"), and sociocultural (the pervasive cultural messaging that thinner is better, teasing or bullying, acculturation, or generational trauma).

Eating disorders are the second-deadliest mental health condition, yet experts say that diagnosis and treatment are largely based on the "SWAG" stereotype: skinny, white, affluent girl. That has prevented Black and marginalized people from getting the help they need. In 2006, for example, one group of researchers found that white women received an eating disorder diagnosis 44 percent of the time and Hispanic women 41 percent, but Black women with identical symptoms were diagnosed only 11 percent of the time. Sizeism, which is discrimination directed against people because of their size, especially related to weight, and fatphobia, which is an irrational fear of or aversion to being fat or being around people who are fat, can also hinder diagnosis and treatment. It is a misconception that people who have eating disorders are thin. People with all body types can have an eating disorder, and that misconception means some people—including men and nonbinary people—are never diagnosed.

Eating disorders can include anorexia nervosa and bulimia, among others. But even disordered eating that doesn't fit the criteria for diagnosis of an eating disorder still presents a risk of health problems. Symptoms may include dieting, anxiety associated with specific foods, chronic weight fluctuations, rigid rules and routines about food and exercise, or using exercise, food restriction, fasting, or purging to counter the "bad food" they consumed; the primary difference between disordered eating and an eating disorder is the severity, frequency, and negative impact of the eating behaviors, not necessarily the behaviors themselves.

Body dysmorphic disorder, a mental health condition in which a person can't stop thinking about one or more perceived defects or flaws in appearance, also causes embarrassment, shame, and anxiety. Often, somebody who suffers from dysmorphia seeks reassurance, repeatedly checks their appearance in the mirror, and experiences challenges to functioning in daily life.

SIGNS, SYMPTOMS, AND RISKS

The National Eating Disorder Association (NEDA) details the signs and symptoms that coaches, parents, and caregivers should look for if they are concerned that an athlete is developing an eating disorder, as well as the health risks that can result from each disorder. These are just a sampling of the associated behaviors and implications—NEDA (nationaleatingdisorders.org) offers online chat, a telephone help line, and texting for more information and support.

Anorexia Nervosa

Signs and symptoms:

- Dramatic weight loss
- Dressing in layers to hide weight loss or stay warm
- Preoccupied with weight, food, calories, and dieting
- Makes frequent comments about feeling fat
- Has constipation, abdominal pain, intolerance to cold, lethargy, or excess energy
- Eats foods in a certain order, excessively chews or rearranges food on the plate
- Makes excuses to avoid group meals
- Needs to "burn off" calories
- Has a rigid exercise routine, despite weather, fatigue, illness, or injury
- Becomes withdrawn, isolated, and secretive
- Has a strong need for control
- Difficulties concentrating and sleeping
- Has abnormal labs like anemia, low thyroid and hormone levels, low potassium, low blood cell counts, slow heart rate
- Dizziness, fainting
- Irregular periods
- Dental problems like enamel erosion, cavities, and tooth sensitivity
- Cuts and calluses on the top of their fingers from inducing vomiting
- Fine hair on the body, thinning of hair on the head

Consequences:

Those who have anorexia nervosa don't have enough nutrients to allow their bodies to function, so the body slows down all of its processes to conserve energy. Electrolyte imbalances are life-threatening, and self-starvation can also lead to cardiac arrest. Long-term, the effects of this disorder lead to bone loss and bone fracture risks much higher than the general population (osteoporosis). Some may have difficulty conceiving children, and others can experience neurological damage like seizures, tingling, or numbness in their hands and feet. One in every five deaths due to anorexia is a result of suicide—it is the highest death rate for any mental health condition.

Bulimia Nervosa

Signs and symptoms:

- Behavior indicates that weight loss and dieting are primary concerns
- Disappearance of large amounts of food in short period of time; empty wrappers and containers
- Frequent trips to the bathroom after meals, signs of vomiting, empty boxes of laxatives or diuretics
- Uncomfortable eating around others
- Has food rituals like only eats particular foods or has eliminated food groups, excessively chews, or doesn't allow foods to touch on a plate
- Skips meals or takes small portions
- Hoards food in hiding places
- Drinks excessive amount of water or noncaloric beverages
- Uses excessive amounts of breath mints, gum, or mouthwash
- Teeth are discolored
- Has cuts on the top of their fingers from inducing vomiting
- Creates schedules to make time for binging and purging
- Looks bloated from fluid retention
- Has extreme mood swings
- Body weight is within the normal range but has noticeable fluctuations up and down
- Has gastrointestinal complaints
- Similar symptoms to anorexia may include abnormal labs, difficulties concentrating and sleeping, fainting and dizziness, intolerance to

THE PRICE SHE PAYS

cold, dental problems, swelling around salivary glands, fine hair on the body, thinning hair on the head, menstrual irregularities
- Often also struggle with self-harm, suicidal thoughts, cutting, substance use, impulsive and risky behaviors

Consequences:
Binging and purging affect the digestive system, leading to electrolyte and chemical imbalances that impact that heart and other organ functions. Many of the same long-term health risks of anorexia also apply to bulimia.

Binge Eating

Most of the signs and symptoms of binge eating mirror those of bulimia, without the purging. The long-term health consequences can include obesity and weight fluctuations. According to NEDA, up to two-thirds of people with binge eating disorder are labeled clinically obese, though people who struggle with it can be any weight.

Compulsive Exercise

Though it isn't a clinical diagnosis, those who struggle with compulsive exercise have several signs and symptoms:

- Their exercise interferes with activities or occurs at inappropriate times, even when injured or ill
- Experiences intense anxiety, depression, irritability, guilt, or distress if unable to exercise
- Find discomfort in rest or inactivity
- Uses exercise to manage emotions
- Purges calories through exercise or need to exercise to give permission to eat
- Exercises in secret
- Overtrains
- Withdraws from friends and family

Consequences:

Similar to eating disorders, those who exercise compulsively suffer from bone density loss (osteoporosis), irregular menstruation, RED-S, overuse injuries, persistent fatigue, increased illnesses, and altered resting heart rate.

Other Specified Feeding or Eating Disorder (OSFED)

This term is used to capture eating disorder pathology that doesn't meet the full criteria for other diagnoses, though it is equally as destructive and debilitating. According to Mariana Prutton, licensed marriage and family therapist in San Francisco, much of what is considered disordered eating could be OSFED if someone is experiencing significant distress or negative physical, mental, and social consequences due to eating behaviors.

UNDERSTANDING COMMON DIAGNOSES AMONG ATHLETES

Female athletes are particularly vulnerable to developing body image and eating disorders, as well as compulsive exercise, which is not a clinical diagnosis, as we mentioned, but causes someone intense anxiety, depression, irritability, or distress when she is unable to exercise. The pressure to perform, develop a certain physique, or even the requirements to wear formfitting or revealing apparel can spur unhealthy, disordered eating, especially if an athlete is part of a team culture that encourages spoken or unspoken rules about body size, weight, and nutrition. All of these variables can result in distorted body image, overtraining, and underfueling.

Disordered eating can be tied to RED-S, which, again, is a syndrome of poor health and declining athletic performance that occurs when athletes do not get enough fuel (calories) to support the energy demands of their lives and training. Any athlete, regardless of gender or ability level, can experience RED-S. Also note that athletes who experience RED-S may not have an eating disorder; they may simply not know or understand how much fuel they need to sustain the level of training they're doing. RED-S can lead to problems with reproductive health, cardiovascular health, immune function, growth, development, and gastrointestinal and metabolic functioning. It can also trigger or exacerbate symptoms of anxiety and depression.

Although all athletes are susceptible to eating disorders, certain sports have a preponderance: those that require weight classes, like rowing, wrestling, and weightlifting, and those that have traditionally valued smaller, leaner physiques to enhance performance, like distance running, gymnastics, figure skating, dance, or diving. Often, female athletes develop body dissatisfaction because of the uniforms they are required to wear, like swimmers and volleyball players, or because they endure critiques about their size and shape. Others feel embarrassed by their muscular appearance, experiencing criticism about their femininity. Individual sports also have more incidences of eating disorders than team sports, probably because the focus is on the singular athlete rather than the collective squad. Other risk factors include family dysfunction, a history of physical or sexual abuse, other trauma, training under a win-at-all-costs coach who utilizes weigh-ins or body composition tests, performance anxiety, or teammates who value thinness. That's a really long way of saying sports can trigger body image and eating disorders in a wide variety of ways, though it's still a combination of factors that lead to a diagnosis.

Maggie Walsh, LMFT, who specializes in eating disorders at Thrive Mental Health in Bend, Oregon, sees patterns with athletes who are seeking help. In endurance sports like cross-country, for example, she's worked with runners who don't actually enjoy the sport but use it as a reason to exercise more without sounding alarm bells to their caregivers. It gives young girls cover because most adults encourage participation in sports for the positive effects they have: skill building, teamwork, physical fitness, healthy habits, and increased self-esteem. "Many clients became three-sport athletes because they were able to have structured time to exercise," Maggie says. "These athletes are using the sport as a means to an end, which results in the disorder."

Then, when an athlete who is already predisposed to or already suffering from anorexia or bulimia finds herself on a team led by a coach who weighs athletes, comments on appearances, and labels food "good" or "bad," it perpetuates the disorders or exacerbates them, Maggie says. Coaches who instruct players to restrict certain food or drinks, or who arbitrarily mandate calorie limits or weight goals, can have a supremely harmful influence on a person who may already be at risk. "Rules" regarding nourishment and food (whether overtly stated or part of the underlying team culture) contribute to the toxicity of a program. Often, body measurements, expectations related to weight or body composition, and rules around what team members are "allowed" to eat are tangible ways to identify dysfunctional leadership or troubled programs.

Lauren entered college diagnosed with anorexia nervosa, for which she had not received treatment. People with anorexia have difficulties maintaining appropriate weight for their height and age, restricting the calories and type of food they eat. They also have an intense fear of gaining weight. Lauren had no intention of playing sports at the small, private, southern university she attended until the cross-country coach spotted her running on campus. His women's team was rebuilding itself due to a plethora of injuries, so he approached her with a scholarship. She liked the idea of joining a team and having organized workouts. For the first year, she was "just a body" to meet participant quotas at competitions. Lauren wasn't on the coach's radar at that point but noticed the way he restricted the team's food choices, walking up and down the bus when they traveled, confiscating any desserts they may have purchased at rest stops. He called sports drinks "empty calories" and never offered them to the team. And he'd limit what the athletes could choose from menus when they were traveling. Lauren recalls how, "even after nationals one year, we went to Dairy Queen with our families and we weren't allowed to get Blizzards."

During the summer, Lauren worked with a group that served impoverished populations in the nearby Appalachian regions. Because of the nature of the work and the conditions, she lost weight. When she returned to practices in the fall, her performance improved, which drew more attention from the coach; she was the second woman ever to make the national meet at the university. But as the pressure mounted, running was no longer fun and Lauren relapsed into calorie restriction. She had told the coach about her history of anorexia, but he dismissed her concerns and her request for help from a dietitian; instead, he praised her performances and told her that she was doing well. "While my eating disorder continued to get worse and worse, my running got better until the end of junior year. I was exercising up to six hours a day, and that eventually took a toll on my body. I was getting a lot of injuries and he'd tell me just to massage them out and keep running. I mean, I was counting the calories in my toothpaste," Lauren says. "I came back senior year weighing eighty pounds, and that was the first time coach was like, 'Oh, you know, maybe something's wrong.'"

At that point, the coach dismissed Lauren from the team and the administration told her to take a medical leave from school while getting treatment. She was promised that her scholarship and spot would remain when she was ready to return. Lauren entered a residential program in another state, then stayed with her parents while recovering. She contacted the coach when she was cleared to return to school, but he stopped communicating with her. "It was like I wasn't good enough anymore and I wasn't worth his time," she says. "He often glorified the perfect body and I never was a calorie counter until I met him."

As is often the case, Lauren has lived with the repercussions of her eating disorder throughout her life. She's now in her forties and still doesn't consider herself in recovery. Her marriage has suffered, and she's been on disability due to having been in and out of treatment for fifteen years. Lauren still limits her food intake on days she doesn't exercise, but all she's allowed to do is light stretching and walking. "I still hear his voice when I have dessert," Lauren says.

Lauren asked for help when she needed it, but her coach never trusted her to know what was best for herself. And when she finally had to leave the team, the coach punished her again by not fulfilling his promise to welcome her back when she was well. "It's still not acceptable, you know," Lauren says. "Society, my family of origin, all those things obviously played a role, but I do believe that my experience with my coach in college played a huge role, too."

IDENTIFYING POTENTIAL PROBLEMS

Rachael Steil, author of *Running in Silence* and founder of the non-profit of the same name, which offers eating disorder awareness and education in the athletic community, began running with her mom in kindergarten, continued competitively through middle school, and then hit a plateau in high school, when the competition got more intense. By that time, she had associated her worth and happiness with running fast, but she hadn't yet cracked the top echelon of girls in Michigan. She saw her sister taking diet pills and realized that maybe exercise wasn't what would change her body, but restricting her diet would. Rachael began limiting food groups, and she lost weight immediately. Her performances improved. She got tips from a running magazine on how to reduce fat, eat "super foods," and limit desserts to once a week.

Soon, Rachael was competing for Aquinas College, in the National Association of Intercollegiate Athletics (NAIA), and seeing a lot of success. But she was hiding her obsession with weight and calorie restriction, often isolating herself from social activities and keeping a rigid eating schedule. Her improved performance only fed her eating disorder, until her body inevitably began to break down with injuries, including a knee injury that sidelined her from running. During that time, she began binge eating, a common pivot for those who have so severely restricted their eating for so long. Binge eating disorder is characterized by recurrent episodes of eating large quantities of food, feeling a loss of control, and then experiencing shame or distress afterward. It's a separate diagnosis from bulimia, which includes behaviors like self-induced vomiting to "undo" or compensate for the effects of binge eating. As Rachael gained more weight, she finally sought help and, in an email to her mom, described everything she had battled over the years.

It still took Rachael eight months to go to treatment, starting with a support group, then working with a therapist and a dietitian, who was also a triathlete and runner. Rachael looped in her coach, who was supportive and encouraged her to put her health ahead of her performance. When she returned to running, she wasn't clocking personal bests, but she was able to remain injury free. Her coach brought up her eating disorder in conversation, which Rachael was grateful for, so she wouldn't have to bring it up herself. Unfortunately, during her senior year, she broke her kneecap, which triggered a relapse. It was time for Rachael to step away from the sport and focus solely on her recovery.

Now, as coach of her former high school cross-country team, Rachael reflects on how important her college coach's support was during that time. He may not have fully understood her eating disorder, but he realized that pushing her to continue to compete would be detrimental to her long-term health—and he worked to alleviate the pressure she felt to perform to her former standards when she returned. "Because he put my health first, I was able to compete for a couple more years," Rachael says.

Rachael's story has been shared a lot within the running world, and for good reason: so many girls and women related to the shame she felt and how she hid the struggles she was going through. People who struggle with eating disorders or disordered eating will often go to great lengths to conceal unhealthy behaviors; that's what makes it so hard for many parents and coaches to identify problems and offer support before they get so serious. During speaking engagements, Rachael displays photos of herself racing at various times during her career and asks the audience to identify which photos were taken during her acute struggles with eating disorders. Often, attendees are surprised to learn that she was in the throes of illness in each photo, not just the one in which she appears smallest. Early intervention leads to better outcomes.

Maggie sees that the parents of many clients didn't realize what they were witnessing with their young athletes. Symptoms like weight loss, amenorrhea (missed periods), or low heart rate, for example, can be explained away by increased fitness. But no teenager (or adult in her child-bearing years, for that matter) should lose their period. Some caregivers give their girls credit for asking them to buy "healthier foods" and avoid bringing sweets home—their discipline and "healthy habits" are applauded. But when entire food groups are eliminated (even sugar, as well as other foods once enjoyed), that change in eating patterns may turn out to be problematic. Use these indicators as a checkpoint for conversations about food. We don't recommend labeling food "good" or "bad" because it leads to issues with eating later on. "Eating disorders are easy to hide," Maggie says. "Parents will say that their daughter is eating all the meals and snacks throughout the day, but they don't actually know. Their daughter will admit that they threw their lunch away at school. That's one reason why so many eating disorders were caught during the pandemic: parents were witnessing the behavior."

Often, parents' interaction with food is replicated by their children. If a parent has a habit of dieting or avoiding "bad" foods like French fries, for example, their children start to recognize that fries are unacceptable, that restricting food is normal, and that a smaller frame is valued. Maggie emphasizes to caregivers that their daughter's eating disorder isn't their fault but encourages them to explore the factors that might need adjustment. You can do everything "right" and your child may still develop a disorder—nobody is to blame. The environment in the home can inadvertently push a girl toward an eating disorder because she's seeking an outlet. Like Jessie Diggins described, she needed to feel in control, because the stress of perfectionism in school and sports was too much.

In the same vein, coaches and teams have distinct cultures around eating food. Teammates' habits can easily rub off on the other athletes in college, where they are living together, traveling together, and

THE PRICE SHE PAYS

sharing meals together. It might be unspoken, but a team that eats salad every night and skips dessert is showing its new members what's expected and appropriate. This behavior is learned the same way kids watch their parents eat and then form a relationship with food that reflects exactly what they observe.

HOW COACHES CAN BETTER NAVIGATE ATHLETE BODY IMAGE, DISORDERED EATING, AND EATING DISORDERS

Mandating body composition testing or constantly weighing athletes is an antiquated and damaging way to coach. If athletes are eating nourishing food, training well, and getting enough recovery, they should never need to worry what the scale says or what their body fat percentage is; it all takes care of itself. Triggering eating disorders by focusing so much attention on weight can lead to devastating outcomes, like suicide, cardiac arrest, or life-long health risks.

So how can coaches help change the culture? Here are a few ideas:

- Think about your own biases related to food, weight, body size, and body image and how these biases influence your work with athletes. What you believe internally will reflect in your engagement with team members. Challenge your beliefs and assumptions about ideal body type and how it's tied to performance; it's helpful to reframe these notions.
- If you suspect that an athlete is struggling, open up a conversation and ask if she has any concerns she'd like to talk about. Often, she will feel relieved that somebody has noticed and is offering help. Eating disorders are notoriously linked to feelings of embarrassment, secrecy, and shame, and eventually, the secret can become too much to bear. The earlier a problem is identified, the more likely treatment will help.

- Emphasize strength, recovery, and mastery of skills instead of appearance or weight. Invite conversations with your athletes about how their bodies feel and what they might need to feel different (better, stronger, less fatigued, and so on). Meet their feedback with curiosity, affirmations, and without judgment.

- Train the staff on the signs and symptoms of eating disorders they should recognize and what to do if they see any. Remember your limits in expertise and refer athletes to professionals who have the training and credentials to help. Host regular check-ins with athletes to normalize discussions about menstrual cycles, RED-S, and concerns about mental and physical well-being. Clearly outline expectations to stay fueled and responses to eating disorders on the team, even when eating disorders are not present.

- Establish relationships with local mental health care providers and registered dietitians who specialize in supporting athletes. Ask them to speak to your team. Create a referral process to ensure access to services for your team, which includes a diverse list of providers who can serve athletes of all identities.

- Give athletes regular access to professionals who can provide accurate information about nutrition and performance so they don't go looking for it themselves and land on unhealthy, outdated, or inaccurate research.

- Talk about the risks and long-term health repercussions associated with underfueling.

- Don't comment about appearance, weight, or food choices, regardless of how innocent or small the comment might seem; even flippant remarks can cause harm.

- Remember that body size and food choices are culturally bound and may also be tied to athlete identity.

- If an athlete develops an eating disorder, work with her medical team to decide how she can remain part of the team. Understand that sports, the community, and her sense of belonging may play a role in her recovery.

TEAM CULTURE, UNSPOKEN RULES, AND
LACK OF EDUCATION

While competing in track and field at Oregon, Katie formed a small group of close friendships. The women helped each other navigate the confusion of such a high-intensity program that had so many unspoken rules, especially about weight and food. Today, as Katie is reflecting so heavily on her experiences while writing this book, she's reached out to some of those women to reminisce. There was that time they went to a football party, and although they didn't drink a sip of alcohol, they still felt like rebels because they were out past the team's 10:00 p.m. curfew. They also recalled what it was like to stop at restaurants as a team and try to figure out what was acceptable to eat. Older teammates would critique the food they chose, they spent many runs talking about what they ate, and they were required to keep food logs that detailed everything down to the number of tortilla chips or peanut M&Ms they consumed.

Katie shared with one of her former teammates how in 2021, six female members of the track and field program came forward, speaking to *The Oregonian*[7] about how the coach required athletes to have regular DEXA scans (imaging tests that measure bone density, muscle mass, and body fat) to measure their body fat percentages, then told them to lower their numbers. One coach even measured body fat with skinfold calipers and kept a record of the results on a spreadsheet, they told the reporters. The athletes described how the practice had led to eating disorders for some—and that a team nutritionist knew that athletes had stopped menstruating, even as they were encouraged to drop weight. All of this led some women to suffer career-ending injuries and others to transfer to other programs. At least one, who had disclosed her eating disorder before arriving at Oregon, went home to recover from a relapse.

In response to that news, Katie's former teammate, now in her late thirties, said, "Isn't that part of being a Division I athlete?" Even all these years later, she was under the impression that an athlete's body was for the property of the university and that an athlete's job was to fulfill the requirements, like lowering her body fat, even if it was an unhealthy suggestion from a coach with no nutrition expertise. But in a way, Katie's friend was right. Too often, that *is* the cost of committing to a college program—just as it had been back when they were athletes, too. Fat-shaming is just part of the agreement, furthering the disconnect so many female athletes have between their minds and bodies. They're conditioned to believe that this is the price they pay for the privilege to compete, whether in distance running or any other sport.

Too often, athletes who muster the courage to talk about their struggles don't receive the response that they need or get shut down or not taken seriously. Alex, an acrobatics and tumbling athlete, for example, was referred to a mental health professional when she started worrying that she was exercising too much and was unsure if she was eating enough to match the demands. The therapist, hired by the athletic department, laughed and told her, "There's nothing to worry about. You're an athlete." Like many young people, Alex didn't know precisely how to explain her unease, but after the talk with the mental health professional, she felt like she had permission to keep doing what she was doing. It's hard to say if the therapist lacked understanding of the situation or wanted a gifted athlete to continue helping the team win. Again, Alex did exactly what she should have done—seek help and support—but was dismissed. When athletes meet with mental health providers, they should expect that the provider will take time to learn about the athlete's concerns, what kind of support they are seeking, and which strategies may have worked or not in the past. Mental health providers should also ask a series of assessment questions, which can help them discover that somebody like Alex had been restricting calories and overexercising. If a mental health provider (especially one hired by the team) does not ask these questions, athletes should seek out a different provider.

Maggie recommends that whether an athlete is the one to broach the topic or it's the parent or coach, the conversation has to revolve around empathy, curiosity, and be free of judgment. Coaches, especially, should realize that they are not experts in nutrition or psychology—but they should also listen to an athlete and approach anybody who they suspect may be struggling. It's not a coach's job to offer opinions about diagnoses or diet. It *is* a coach's job to make sure the athlete has access to the appropriate professionals who can offer help. The same goes for parents: Early intervention is crucial, so if you sense a problem, start with a primary care provider, reach out to a therapist, or make an appointment with a dietitian. "Ask your child directly if they think they are struggling with an eating disorder," Maggie says. "Do not just let it go. Early intervention like residential treatment or partial hospitalization or intensive outpatient programs can feel extreme, but teens get better when they get out of their environment. It will be a lot of work, but adolescents get better."

The NCAA has no policy regarding how programs should train coaches on RED-S, body image, and eating disorders—or how to approach subjects like fueling and nutrition. It does offer guidelines and warns that coaches have "considerable influence" when it comes to these issues—and that the more conflict and less support there is between coach and athlete, the higher the risk of an athlete developing an eating disorder. Eating disorders have, indeed, become entrenched in sport culture and the lack of protocol for how coaches can help athletes succeed without encouraging these conditions is a problem. The fact that so many are still correlating body size and appearance with performance perpetuates the cycle.

Nobody denies that body composition is a factor in how an athlete performs, but not every athlete performs best at her lowest weight. And, in fact, often a lower weight sacrifices other important functions like muscular strength, power, endurance, and aerobic capacity. We often mistake low body weight and small size with health (sizeism), which is not true for anybody, including athletes. The coach who encourages open discussions about how and why female bodies change and celebrates the factors that lead to success—like teamwork, enthusiasm, and dedication—ultimately have the better results.

Chapter Nine

UNDERSTANDING SUICIDE
AND SELF HARM

Although sports can offer some protection from suicide
and self-harm, athletes also face unique risks due
to their participation.

---

*Note: If you are thinking about harming yourself or attempting sui-
cide, call 988, the national Suicide & Crisis Lifeline, which provides
free and confidential emotional support to people in suicidal crisis
or emotional distress twenty-four-hours-a-day, seven-days-a-week in
the United States.*

Katie Meyer was the only girl in her preschool class of fourteen children. Her dad, Steve Meyer, remembers how compelled his daughter felt to keep up with all those boys, always jumping off playground
equipment, climbing trees, trying to beat them in sprint races at recess.
From a young age, Katie had a swagger about her. "A little spitfire,"
Steve says of his middle child. "She was so fun. She had that curiosity
and that glint of mischievousness. Her wheels were always spinning a
little bit like that." It wasn't long until she found a way to channel that
energy, through soccer.

From the time she started on the local youth team, where she quickly graduated to club level, she discovered her sacred ground: in the goal. "Goalkeeper just fit her personality," says Gina, Katie's mother. "Away from soccer, she loved talent shows. In second grade, she closed the talent show singing Kelly Clarkson's 'A Moment Like This.'" According to Gina, Katie's love of performing may explain why she was drawn to the position. "Kind of like, 'This is my stage, enjoy the show.' She played with such a flare and panache to her."

During high school, she took online classes while traveling for elite tournaments and camps—and in the process she learned how to prioritize the demands of rigorous athletics and academics, her parents say. When it came time to pick a college, she chose Stanford University, where she was recognized as the MVP of the 2019 College Cup championship game against the University of North Carolina, which Stanford won in a penalty shootout, thanks to two big saves by Katie. She went on to become a team captain in 2020 and 2021. And along with her soccer stardom, she served as a resident assistant and was awarded fellowships and scholar opportunities.

By her senior year, Katie had applied to Stanford Law School and was hoping to either attend or defer, depending on whether she entered the draft for the National Women's Soccer League. But one unusual source of stress that year was causing her a lot of anxiety. She was facing disciplinary action from Stanford's Office of Community Standards. In August 2021, Katie had allegedly spilled coffee on another Stanford athlete, a football player who had been accused of sexually assaulting one of Katie's younger teammates. (Stanford says its Title IX office found "the criteria for moving forward with an investigation were not met.") For months afterward, she had feared that the repercussions of the incident would derail her ambitious postgraduation goals.

In her formal statement to the Office of Community Standards in November 2021, Katie wrote,[1] in part: "female athletes know that one mistake can ruin everything. My whole life I've been terrified to make any mistakes. No alcohol, no speeding tickets, no A- marks on my report cards. Everything had to be perfect to get in and stay at Stanford. I suffer from anxiety and perfectionism, as so many female athletes do. We know all too well that in professional settings women have everything to lose and have to work twice as hard to prove that they are qualified and professional, and any mistake is magnified, any attitude of assertiveness is demonized."

Late at night on February 28, 2022, three months shy of graduation, Katie received a six-page disciplinary charge letter that, in part, put her status as a Stanford student and athlete into question and placed her diploma on hold. On March 1, Katie Meyer, age twenty-two, was found dead in her dorm room. An autopsy confirmed she had died by suicide.

"In that moment, I think she was looking at life through a little straw and she couldn't see anything else—like everything was going to come crashing down after working so hard," Gina says. "She couldn't see anything on the outside. It was one dark, desperate moment that I truly believe, if she could have taken it back, she would've. Had she gone for a walk, had somebody knocked on her door, had she made a phone call. I think anything could have changed that moment." Steve and Gina Meyer say that they never identified any distressing signs or symptoms in Katie before she died. In fact, they had spoken to her over FaceTime earlier that evening and remember her being in great spirits that night, making travel plans for spring break and confirming a campus visit with her dad later that week. After recovering from an injury, she was ready to start training again and wanted her father to help jumpstart her comeback. "We didn't have any of those glaring red flags, so it was beyond shocking," Steve says.

It's often confusing and disorienting for loved ones to reconcile what they witnessed before their family member died by suicide. In Katie Meyer's case, self-described anxiety about perfectionism didn't present to the outside world as suicidality. Her enthusiasm about the future seemed like a sign that she was safe, which is a common belief among those who have had a loved one die by suicide, though often not true.

The impulsiveness of suicide can result in surprise and shock for those who knew the person who died.

DEEP DESPAIR

Katie Meyer was one of at least five female collegiate athletes who died by suicide in the spring of 2022. The NCAA doesn't keep public data on such fatalities, but a 2015 study[2] found that college athletes overall had a lower rate of suicide than the rest of the college population. In some ways, sports can protect people from mental health struggles; as we've mentioned before, physical activity, exercise, and the sense of community and belonging help reduce symptoms of depression and boost self-esteem. That said, one study by the Centers for Disease Control and Prevention (CDC) found that the protective aspects apply more for male athletes than female. Participation in sports can also increase the chances somebody could experience bullying, hazing, abuse, and substance use, all risk factors for suicide. Concussions may also be linked to suicidal thoughts and depression. Generally, for all the benefits we know to be true about sports, plenty of factors are also contributors to mental health crises, whether symptoms preexisted outside of participation or have been exacerbated by athletics.

In the general population, US suicide rates increased in 2021, following a two-year decline, according to the CDC.[3] The rates among young people and people of color were worse than other demographics. Between 2018 and 2021, the suicide rate rose 19.2 percent among Black people, and for Black people ages ten to twenty-four, it increased 36.6 percent. Among all people ages twenty-five to forty-four, suicide rates increase 5 percent, with American Indian or Alaska Native people experiencing the starkest spike, increasing by 26 percent. At the time the statistics were released in February 2023, experts guessed that the racial disparities were because these communities were disproportionately affected by the impacts of the COVID-19 pandemic, like job loss, social isolation, financial trouble, and barriers to health care, as well the deaths of a loved ones. Generational trauma and racism could also factor in.

In February 2023, the CDC also reported that the demographic that fared the worst in 2021 across nearly all measures of mental health, including suicidal thoughts and behaviors, were girls and LGBQ youth (lesbian, gay, bisexual, or questioning, as defined in this study). The Youth Risk Behavior Survey,[4] which examines health behaviors and experiences among US high school students, found that youth mental health has declined overall, especially among girls: nearly 30 percent seriously considered attempting suicide in 2021, a 60 percent increase from ten years ago. Half of LGBQ students had recently experienced poor mental health, and more than 22 percent had attempted suicide. In a 2020 study published by the *Journal of Adolescent Health*,[5] transgender and nonbinary youth were up to 2.5 times more likely to experience symptoms of depression, seriously consider suicide, and attempt suicide, compared to their cisgender LGBQ peers, because of the mistreatment, harm, and biases of society that increase hopelessness.

Athletes have their own risk factors, too. Somebody who is feeling disconnected, whether because of an injury or a performance issue—or, possibly in Katie Meyer's case, the threat of losing her team, her place at the university, and her pursuit of future endeavors—may well contribute to the distress. Thoughts of suicide can also be triggered when an athlete loses a sense of identity, like when they are cut from a team or retiring, for example.

Suicide risk increases as a sense of hope decreases. It, like many mental health conditions, is an intensely individual experience, and at the heart of it is deep despair. But we know that the vast majority of people contemplating suicide don't actually want to die. They're seeking an end to intense mental or physical pain and suffering. Suicide is an escape, a temporary relief; often, a death by suicide is triggered by an immediate crisis that may have led the person to feel humiliation, shame, or loss.

Emily was cut from the large southern university swim team to which she had been recruited after a new coaching staff arrived. It was devastating, but she relied heavily on her faith during that time and remembers attending a church service where the pastor preached about how precious our time is. He compared time to a gift card—use it wisely, he said. As she exited the church, she cried and told her room-mate, "I'm so tired. I'm so worn out. I feel like I want to throw my gift card away," Emily says.

The first time Emily had suicidal thoughts was when she was sixteen years old, but this time those thoughts were more intense. A friend and a person who worked at the church took her to the hospital that night. She begged them not to call her parents—she didn't want them to worry. After falling asleep in a chair in the hospital, she was checked in at 2:00 a.m. by the coroner. As it turns out, in the state where the hospital was located, it's the coroner who signs mental health patients in for seventy-two hours of care, deciding if they are a threat to themselves or others. (And to be clear, we don't think it's great for mental health patients to be evaluated by a coroner.)

The next morning, Emily was strapped in and transported by ambu-lance to an in-patient psychiatric hospital two hours away. By this time her mother had been contacted, but Emily had no idea where to tell her she was being taken because she didn't know. Her father found the facility and checked into a nearby hotel. Her parents had power of attorney, but it held no power in the behavioral health setting. She was in treatment with people who had severe mental health conditions, though she did not have the same diagnosis as any of them. She spoke with her parents by phone for forty minutes each day, until she was released six days later. "I never envisioned something like that happen-ing to me," Emily says. "The hospital ended up being helpful in the end when I could relate to some other people who were similar to me who were there. I kind of did, in a way, get a renewed sense of life because I wanted to fight as hard as I could to not end up in this situation ever again." During that time, Emily's parents reiterated each day that they were there for her, that they'd all get through it, and that they loved her. "I did feel my symptoms dissipate . . . those suicidal thoughts, it was as if they had vanished after those six days," she says. "But there were definitely moments that I was like, 'I'm never going to swim again. Am I even going to finish my degree? Is this going to taint the rest of my life?' I was worried about that."

The reality is that in some areas of the United States, medical practices when it comes to mental health are antiquated. Emily's experience is not unique. These practices tend to isolate people amid their most intense needs for support and miss how imperative relational care is. Emily needed her family, and like any other person struggling with mental health, she deserved to have them integrated into her care. We allow somebody admitted to the ER with a broken leg to have friends or family members stay with them while they receive care, so why wouldn't we afford that to anybody else? What tends to happen in medical settings is not trauma-informed and therefore unhelpful for long-term recovery. It can keep people from wanting to seek support, resulting in longer suffering because their options for care are limited.

It is possible—and even common—to help someone transition from suicidal thoughts to a place of healing and hope, beginning by asking direct questions (and not all questions at once): How are you coping with what's going on in your life? Have you had any thoughts about killing yourself? Have you been thinking about how you might do this? Have you had some intention of acting on these thoughts? Despair, impulse, and access to a lethal means is a deadly combination, and the more reports we hear of suicide among athletes, the more people begin to feel like it's an effective way to end suffering. When athletes feel like a burden to their coaches, parents, or teammates, it can increase their distress. Opening up a conversation with somebody who is going through stressful times and offering to help that person seek assistance can change the outcome dramatically. The same questions should be utilized regardless of the person's age, though increased monitoring of youth can be useful.

And if you're talking with somebody who is actively seeking a way to die, immediately take lethal means away, such as firearms and medication. The most important way to offer help to somebody is to remain curious. We know that we can't fully understand what other people are experiencing or feeling, so offering a list of "all the things they have to live for" isn't the best way to be supportive. Instead, make sure the athlete understands that her emotions are valid and that she is allowed to express them. Compassion and safety are crucial, so take her somewhere that she feels safe, give her a break, and sit with her through those tough moments.

With the help of a licensed mental health practitioner, caregivers should try to talk with the athlete about what is underlying their loss of hope. How does the culture of the team or the expectations of the season play a role? How does the athlete feel about her relationship with the coaching staff? Are aspects of her role as an athlete contributing to feelings of depression, stress, anxiety, or trauma? One athlete told us she doesn't want anyone to ask her *why* she is having suicidal thoughts. Although we all want to know what is causing somebody so much pain, it's a deeply personal question and it's not necessary to know why. Some may not even know or have an answer. Instead, rely on compassion instead of inquisition. Clearly state that you understand your athlete is struggling and ask how you can help.

RECOGNIZING SIGNS OF POSSIBLE SUICIDAL THOUGHTS AMONG ATHLETES

Athletes often don't fit the typical description of somebody suffering from suicidal thoughts. They still go to class, study, attend team meetings, train for hours every day, and travel to competitions, among the other important aspects of life, like eating and sleeping. To the untrained eye, they often look as though they're healthy, highly ambitious humans. Moreover, because athletes have become so conditioned to masking emotional pain, recognizing symptoms and treating them early becomes impossible.

The signs of trouble for athletes can be subtle, but those closest to them, like teammates, trainers, and coaches, are in the best position to notice shifts and ask questions. Here are some symptoms to watch, according to the NCAA:

- Talking, writing, or thinking about death
- An increase in impulsive, aggressive, or reckless behavior
- Increased substance use
- Social withdrawal from friends and teammates
- Dramatic mood swings
- Mood shifts from despair to calm
- Unexplained performance dips in sport and/or academics
- Sleep difficulties and fatigue
- Overuse injuries
- Changes in appetite and/or weight

WHAT LEADS TO SELF-HARM

Self-harm, which is intentional harm to the body, is widely misunderstood and stigmatized. Professionals now name it "non-suicidal self-injury," or NSSI, to make clear that the behavior is not suicidal. It's often a coping mechanism, and it's strongly linked to trauma, including childhood sexual trauma. Other reasons for self-harm can include coping with big or overwhelming emotions, managing upsetting thoughts, trying to feel less numb, or expressing pain when you can't find the words to express it. The most common forms of self-harm are cutting the skin, subdermal tissue scratching, burning oneself, banging the head, or punching things or oneself. The average age of onset of self-harm is thirteen, which may be due to the intensity of hormones during puberty. It doesn't tend to discriminate, either—research doesn't show a difference in rates of self-harm due to gender, race, or ethnicity, though the condition is understudied.

Self-harm generally serves two purposes: numbing when emotions are too intense and/or activating emotions when you're feeling numb. It is not a suicide gesture; it's actually sometimes a way to resist or escape suicidal thoughts (though, somewhat confusingly, a person can be using self-harm to cope and, simultaneously, also be suicidal). Self-harm can produce a physiological sensation that actually helps that person feel better—in fact, the brain releases dopamine, mimicking an opioid high—and the more somebody cuts, the stronger rush they feel, the more they may cut again. It can also help somebody feel a sense of control or create visible wounds that match the internal hurt.

Suicide and self-harm don't have a single cause; they're the result of a complex array of factors in an individual's life and can vary by gender, age, and ethnicity. Family life seems to play a big role. Growing up in an environment of child abuse, neglect, or having caregivers ignore or reject a child's emotions, or having poor attachment relationships, for example, can all contribute. Self-harm, like many behaviors that people don't understand, still carries stigma, which of course makes it difficult for anybody to ask for help. But just like any other health issue, self-harm is a symptom of an underlying problem.

Rhonda, for example, a highly recruited softball player, came to compete for a prominent program from a tumultuous childhood. Her father was physically, sexually, and emotionally abusive and controlled her every move as a young player. Whereas the community saw him as a dedicated parent, Rhonda kept his behavior a secret while her mother did nothing to protect her.

Rhonda's coping mechanism was cutting, which allowed her to temporarily release emotional pain. Going to college was an opportunity to escape her abuser and find a fresh start. But as one of the newest members of the team, she was isolated and no longer the star (a hurdle many college athletes face). She secretly engaged in more self-harm to cope until a teammate realized what was going on. Rhonda's coaches immediately referred her to a treatment program and didn't allow her to continue playing. The help she received was pivotal, but Rhonda had to shed her identity as a collegiate athlete forever. She never competed again.

For athletes, having dysfunctional or invalidating relationships with coaches or teammates can lead some to self-harm. The former teen track star Mary Cain, for example, said she began self-harming while experiencing public body-shaming and other forms of emotional abuse from her coach, Alberto Salazar. It can manifest even if the athlete's family life is stable and healthy, as Mary has described her own.

Once, when Tiffany was presenting at a national conference, two hundred fellow therapists showed up to hear her lecture about self-harm. So many of her clients had told her how therapists often got it wrong, so it was an opportunity to help more people in her profession get it right. At the end of her talk, a prominent male professor shared that in his experience, self-harm was all about attention. He didn't offer further insight, and he probably wasn't expecting Tiffany's response: She agreed. People who are suffering want and need attention. And that's a mental health practitioner's job—to provide the attention, care, and under-standing they need to make the pain stop. Tiffany often says to think of those moments as opportunities for connection, rather than attention.

Cat, the swimmer who started her collegiate swimming career at a southern Power 5 program, scratched her face and hit herself as a way to cope with intense scrutiny and lack of support. In her teen years, the behavior escalated to cutting. In her youth, she sometimes hoped that somebody would see the cuts on her body as a physical manifestation of her suffering, but even though she wore a swimsuit almost daily, almost nobody noticed what was happening. When she moved on to college, Cat's condition became severe. Her coach consulted the psychiatrist, and the psychiatrist mishandled the situation. She asked Cat to take off her jacket, grabbed her arm, and made Cat look at her wounds, only to declare that Cat didn't need stitches (insinuating that the situation wasn't severe). The psychiatrist's tone was shaming, accusatory, scary, and didn't follow professional, trauma-informed protocol. "My mentally ill brain just heard, 'I can go deeper next time,'" Cat says. "For me, before I self-harmed, it was for a release, but in my head, I thought maybe somebody would help me. Afterward, I was so ashamed I didn't want anybody to know."

Gwen, who played soccer at a mid-Atlantic Division II university, hid her cutting from view by only self-harming on her ribs and thighs. She started self-harming during the stress of finals week her first semester, after what she felt was a poor performance during soccer season, as a way to cope with the transition to college athletics and academics. "It became a frequent occurrence when I would slip into numbness and this would happen when I didn't feel good enough, when I felt like a disappointment, which would become a regular thing," Gwen says.

Her head coach never knew about her struggles. He didn't create an environment that felt safe to talk about mental health; Gwen believed if she told him, she'd lose any chance of playing. Eventually, during her final two years, she confided in an assistant coach and the team's trainer. As it turned out, the trainer's office became a place where somebody offered reassurance, care, and concern. The trainer also provided accountability, making sure Gwen went to therapy, took her medication, got enough sleep, and remained healthy. This attention and care were instrumental in her recovery. "No one essentially got anything wrong, but I wish my head coach had created an atmosphere where it was safe to talk about mental health with no judgment," Gwen says. "There were small comments made that reinforced that I was making the right decision in keeping it to myself."

We're glad that Gwen found a connection with somebody on staff who could help. We also believe that if all coaches and staff created an environment that allowed and encouraged athletes to express their concerns, help could be offered more quickly. That would result in less suffering and increased performance, too. We know that mental health conditions are treatable, but not if athletes remain fearful that their needs and careers may be dismissed by the people in power.

HOW TO INTERVENE IF SOMEONE NEEDS HELP

Every program should have a suicide prevention protocol in place, especially on college campuses, where the coach will likely receive a call and need to intervene. Here are some dos and don'ts when it comes to helping an athlete in crisis:

- If an athlete has confided that she has intent or a plan to attempt suicide, take it seriously, no matter what—never assume such a declaration is "for attention."
- Have the names and phone numbers of licensed mental health practitioners on hand, including the student health center, campus counseling centers, local services, psychiatric emergency centers, and after-hours resources. Make a list of all options available at any time of day or night and look for people who understand sports and athletes.
- Make sure the athlete is not left alone—she should have someone with her until an evaluation by a licensed mental health practitioner is complete.
- Remember that the athlete's health care team should determine whether she should return to training and competition. Depending on the situation, it might be beneficial to treatment—though for others, it might exacerbate symptoms. Athletes should participate in this discussion, letting their support team know what feels best and possible for them. Give athletes agency in these decisions.
- Coaches should always show compassion, empathy, and listen to their athletes, but also understand their limits.

STEPS TOWARD SAVING LIVES

Since their daughter's death, the Meyers have started an organization called Katie's Save, a movement to implement a system at colleges and universities nationwide that would allow students the option to designate an advocate who the institution has permission to contact if a student is involved in a situation where they may need guidance or support. In Katie's case, her advocate would have received notice that she was dealing with a disciplinary action and could have reached out and offered help, empathy, or just lent an ear.

Bella, a soccer player at a large university in New England, says she used self-harm to cope with her student-athlete experience. "I was cutting daily just to feel something, compared to being numb and emotionless and depressed," she says. During her sophomore year, Bella attempted suicide after a championship game. Her teammate and best friend intervened, taking her to a hospital where she remained for a week. Up until that game, Bella had been cutting herself and having suicidal thoughts as she was struggling with her confidence. "I felt I was at wit's end—my athletic performance was lacking and my whole identity was associated with soccer, how I would perform, or how much I would play," she says. "I was tired of the constant mental battle with myself, and I wanted it all to end. My best friend saved my life that day and that is the reason I am alive."

While her coaches were aware of Bella's struggles, they didn't know the extent of her distress. Since she was released from the hospital, she's found them supportive of her mental health, feeling a sense that they care about her outside of her performance on the field. She hesitated for so long to tell them about her challenges because she "felt stupid and weak," she says. "I feared that they would not care or see me differently than the person I am . . . I regret not getting therapy sooner and regret not asking for help earlier on, before things got so overwhelming to where I felt I was at the point of no return."

Now Bella has found some healing in journaling, where she can write about any of her emotions or experiences where she knows she won't be judged. When she feels waves of anxiety, she tries deep breathing exercises. In other words, she has found healthier ways of coping than self-harm. "No sport or academic performance is worth your life,"

Bella says. "You can't have a job, play the game you love, or anything if you aren't alive." As a person of color, Bella felt it was common for her and other athletes of color to not seek help or support when they needed it. Her university, she says, is trying to hire a staff that includes more diverse representation, which can make it easier for athletes of color to connect with them. Having the option to talk with a therapist who fully understands your race and ethnicity can also encourage more people to seek treatment.

"I am Hispanic, but we only have one Black person on our team. That has been the case as an athlete—there will be like two people of color and it's hard to open up about how we feel when things come up," Bella says. "We brought it up to the athletic department and they've worked really hard to change things. They strive to make changes for the betterment of student athletes."

What's important is that even though Bella had experienced significant mental health needs, she felt seen and heard as an athlete. She even offered feedback to the athletic department, which sparked change. It goes to show, yet again, that athletes know what they need and are better poised to succeed when the people in power are available and interested in what they have to say.

Often, in the throes of stress, anxiety, or depression, it might be too hard for that student to pick up the phone, send a text, or write an email asking for help. And sometimes athletes are intimidated by the power imbalances they encounter, whether it's a coach, a professor, or the institution itself. But having someone, whether it's a parent, a sibling, another family member, or a trusted friend, already looped in and checking in could make a difference.

As they've talked to more experts and college leaders, the Meyers have also identified other areas that could improve. College campuses work in silos, so if an athlete is injured, had surgery, and is falling behind academically, it's unlikely that the athletics department, her academic advisor, her medical team, and coaches will communicate with each other. Meanwhile, that athlete is feeling exhausted, overwhelmed, and completely disconnected from her routine and her people. It's a recipe for disaster. A more holistic approach to students' well-being would not only enhance the experience but also potentially prevent the worst outcomes.

Athletics departments at every level could also require trainers, coaches, and staff to undergo suicide prevention and intervention training. Free online training (with course completion certificates) is offered through the Columbia Severity Rating Scale, or the American Psychological Association lists other psychological first aid training courses. Learning to identify the signs of distress among athletes and how to take action is mental health first aid, which is just as critical as other required courses, like "regular" First Aid, CPR, and AED certifications. It would go a long way toward changing the way people involved in athletic systems talk about mental health and foster cultures that embrace those conversations without making athletes feel like they might suffer consequences for acknowledging their conditions.

Chapter Ten

UNDERSTANDING SUBSTANCE USE

The reasons why female athletes use alcohol or other substances are varied but not widely talked about.

The day Abby Wambach saw her mug shot on the ESPN ticker in 2016 was the day she realized that alcohol use had "done me dirty." She was newly retired from professional soccer and separating from her first wife. While moving her belongings, including her Olympic gold medals and world championship awards, from her home, she drank. And she drove. She was pulled over, arrested, and spent a night in a Portland, Oregon, jail. The next day, with reporters and photographers camped outside of her ex-wife's home, she was inside watching ESPN, her mugshot staring back at her on the screen. "I thought my life was over. I thought everything that I had spent my life building and doing—playing soccer, traveling the world, fighting for women's equality—I now was going to be put in the category of canceled," Abby said during a March 2023 podcast episode of *We Can Do Hard Things*, with her wife, Glennon Doyle.[1]

Abby enrolled in a diversion program that required her to remain alcohol and drug free for one year, take random drug tests, and receive court-ordered therapy. The significant legal repercussions she would face if she chose to consume alcohol and prescription drugs like Vicodin, Ambien, and Adderall, came as a relief, she said. "That's all I needed. I needed that so much. I needed somebody to be like, 'Can't do it anymore or else you'll be in jail,'" Abby said on the podcast. "And I needed every second of the shame that ESPN ticker gave me. I needed all of the wake-up call this opportunity gave me . . . to actually see what was happening in my life."

Abby went on to write *Forward: A Memoir*,[2] in which she revealed that she had started drinking as a teenager, a habit that soon evolved into a way to split herself "from soccer player into normal person." During offseasons and in between intense training and competition blocks, she also used substances to numb heartbreaks and cope with the pressure of being a gay athlete in a high-profile marriage that was coming to an end. "I always was struggling with, 'Do I think I'm drinking too much?' and I would do it for short periods of time because soccer . . . protected me from that part of myself," Abby said during the podcast. "It was like this safety mechanism that was in place."

Abby is one of the few female athletes who has spoken openly about substance use. In fact, in our conversations with all of our focus groups, along with dozens of other female athletes, and even as we put out a few public calls for others to discuss substance-use disorder, we didn't find many who were willing to talk about it. Research released in 2023 by Penn State University showed that fewer than 11 percent of all women (not just athletes) with a substance-use disorder received treatment in 2019.[3] The study analyzed responses of 461 women to the National Survey on Drug Use and Health between 2015 and 2019, finding that across economic, educational, and cultural lines, women did not seek treatment because of stigma, logistics like transportation and childcare, and lack of perceived need or readiness.

Substance-use disorders (SUDs) are chronic—and treatable (according to the 2021 National Survey on Drug Use and Health, seven in ten adults who have ever had a substance use problem consider themselves to be recovering or in recovery[4])—illnesses marked by a problematic pattern of use and loss of control over the use of substances like alcohol, cannabis, hallucinogens, inhalants, opioids, sedatives, stimulants, or tobacco, leading to impairments in health and social function. Anybody, regardless of age, race, gender, or socioeconomic status can be affected by SUDs and, in fact, one in seven Americans aged twelve or older reports experiencing this kind of disorder, according to the Centers for Disease Control and Prevention.

Alcohol is the most common substance that teens experiment with, and girls between ages twelve and seventeen have a slightly higher rate of use than boys, according to the National Institute on Drug Abuse. Women have reported using drugs to control weight, fight exhaustion, cope with pain, and self-treat mental health conditions. Substance use is a common way for a person to feel different. For example, alcohol disrupts the brain's communication pathways, which lowers inhibition and allows people to "get out of their own head," triggers more dopamine, and produces feelings of pleasure. Opioids block pain signals from the brain to the body and also trigger the release of dopamine. Athletes often want to feel different, whether it's to speed up or cope with injury recovery, ease anxiety or depression, or, like Abby, feel like they have a "normal life" outside of the hyperfocus of sport. Substance use is a reliable way to change how you feel, and it often has such a powerful effect, some people use it again and again because it becomes psychologically addictive.

Bella, the soccer player at a university in New England, says that for her teammates and other athletes, drinking on the weekends helps them feel less "like a robot." But she doesn't sense that anybody pressures anybody else to indulge if they don't want to. Offseason benders are normal, she says, and it's often hard to stop when training rolls around again. "Substance use is a social decision when the team goes out," Bella says. "Some people don't do it, and nobody holds it against them, but the majority of the people do and it's part of a normal college experience, versus just being in season and working hard all the time and in all the ways."

For the athletes we work with, the compulsion that drives them to compete and perform is often linked to the addictive part of their brains (their reward circuit). When participating in athletics becomes less rewarding or they step away from it, they often feel an intense need to fulfill that compulsion; in other words, they go through a form of withdrawal, like what happens when a heavy substance user stops using drugs or alcohol. Often, talented athletes don't know how to moderate their substance use well because they are accustomed to doing everything at full capacity, so early intervention with young people is beneficial.

The statistics show that substance-use disorders likely occur at lower rates among athletes than in the general population, and that their incidence is on the decline. In 2017, the NCAA's most recent survey of its athletes, 39 percent reported binge drinking (having four or more drinks in one sitting), down from 51 percent of female athletes who reported binge drinking in 2009,[5] and the statistics show that NCAA athletes in all three divisions are using marijuana and amphetamines at lower rates than the general student population.

Competing at a high level appears somewhat protective against SUDs in some areas of sports, outside of using performance-enhancing drugs. But athletes tend to become more susceptible or vulnerable to SUDs at stressful junctures in their careers, like during injuries and when they retire (see more about the mental health implications of retirement in chapter 13). And for college athletes, drinking and using other substances are often a rite of passage; in fact, many athletes find campuses an abstinence-hostile environment, a term coined by experts in the collegiate recovery field.[6] When substance use is part of the culture, it's difficult to resist the social influences and expectations to fit in. One NCAA Division I swimmer remembers her recruiting visit to a big-name program, when she was taken to a party. At first, she refused a drink, until her hostess remarked, "On this team, you drink."

AN OUNCE OF PREVENTION?

In a 2012 NCAA survey of twenty-one thousand athletes across all divisions and sports, 89 percent said that coaches and administrators had talked about expectations regarding drinking and substance use, but a third of the women wanted more discussions among their teams.[7] Often, the conversations with young people on this subject are punitive, which we've found does not work. Older generations will remember the 1980s "Just Say No" campaign, urging the youth of America to "just say no" to drugs and alcohol (as if it were so simple). Instead, we've found that having meaningful and transparent conversations about consuming substances likely leads to better understanding. Again, it's a matter of normalizing and naming such topics so they are less taboo.

The stigma around these discussions stems, at least in part, around misconceptions about who struggles with substance use. For example, when we're young, adults point to people they don't want us to become— those who are unhoused or who go to bars by themselves—as cautionary tales about the consequences of using alcohol or drugs. In these moments, however, we are disregarding the facts about substance use— framing it as a simple choice, when in fact it can be a difficult illness. The conversation about substance use can also become racist and discriminatory: we criminalize use and incarcerate communities under the guise of a "drug crisis" and policing the "bad guys." But can you imagine if we discussed cancer as an issue of spending too much time in a "bad" neighborhood? This doesn't mean that people aren't responsible for their behavior, but we shouldn't miss the nuance of the illness itself—the powerful nature of craving and withdrawal are medically induced with our brains and bodies. We've decided as a culture that drinking in college is a rite of passage and that having a glass of wine every night is an acceptable way to unwind. But in the end, we're all trying to feel different or take the edge off in the same way.

The desire to use alcohol or substances is normal; we're socialized throughout college and adulthood to toast accomplishments, to destress, and to catch up with friends over a drink. It's okay to normalize attitudes athletes have and allow them to come to conclusions about use together instead of policing it, as well as recognize that some people also don't want to drink or use substances for a variety of reasons. Instead of pointing to big-name athletes who "ruined their lives" with excessive substance use and telling young people, "Don't be like them—you'll lose everything," suggest that they find alternative ways to connect to each other or other outlets to release stress. Research proves that fear tactics and threats of punishment don't work.

Michelle Pitts, PhD, conducted a 2018 study, "Athletes' Perceptions of Their Head Coach's Alcohol Management Strategies and Athlete Alcohol Use,"[8] measuring three ways that coaches commonly use: enforcement (clearly defined rules about alcohol use and explicit consequences for violations); conditional leniency (coach is permissive or accepting of drinking under certain circumstances and lacks general discouragement); and concerned communication (coach talks about the consequences of alcohol use, discusses safe drinking, and is aware of athlete drinking attitudes and behaviors; creates a comfortable and approachable climate). Pitts asked 897 collegiate female softball players from sixty-three NCAA teams what methods worked best and found that higher concerned communication and lower conditional leniency resulted with less athlete alcohol use, while enforcement had no effect (again, "just say no" doesn't work).

It's common for teams to designate their own rules and norms related to alcohol and other substance consumption. It becomes part of the culture. One acrobatics and tumbling athlete told us that members were not allowed to drink while wearing any team gear or while traveling for competition (even if a teammate was meeting with family members separately for a meal). The coaches decided that athletes could have one night of drinking per week if they didn't have a practice the next morning, which usually narrowed it down to Fridays. Another athlete, a pole-vaulter, said her team set expectations about drinking and marijuana use during meetings.

Teammates often keep each other accountable, especially during competitive seasons, whether it's "no drinking twenty-four hours before a game" or "no drinking during the season," the athletes we spoke with agree that it's usually up to the group to look out for each other. "From my point of view, each sport sort of has their own cultural expectations around drinking that have been formed over the years and kind of enforced at the seniority level," the pole-vaulter says.

Putting the responsibility on peers at the high school and college levels to notice if a teammate is struggling with a substance-use disorder is a big ask, however. Madeline* was a key member of a national championship-bound acrobatics team who joined her teammates for a night out in a town where they wouldn't be recognized. Drinking with first-year athletes was a violation of team rules, and they didn't want to get caught. But that night, Madeline fell and hit her head, causing a concussion. Knowing that she'd be asked questions that would force her to admit how she'd sustained the injury, she didn't tell anyone about it and went out drinking again on Saturday. It wasn't until Wednesday that she had to seek help because her symptoms were so bad. But after the team medical staff found out she had broken a team rule and lied about it, she was pulled from practice and the upcoming meet.

The big piece of information that the medical staff missed or ignored was that Madeline was a known heavy drinker among her teammates, beyond the "typical" college student's behavior. Their goal was to get this star to return to competition quickly. A secondary concern was the violation of team rules. What the staff didn't offer was support or intervention for substance use. Because she had been caught with teammates, they had to enforce the rules, but the focus was on getting her back on mat and winning the national championship, which would boost the university's reputation. All while turning away from obvious signs of a major substance use issue right in front of them.

What might athletic staff and caregivers notice as signs of a possible substance-use disorder? Athletes who struggle to cut down on use, despite stating their desire or intention to do so. Somebody who breaks team rules around drugs and alcohol, who is late to functions, or whose grades are declining. A player who struggles interpersonally—maybe they isolate more or get into arguments with their teammates. Somebody who gets frustrated if others suggest they might have a problem or feels guilty after they use.

TALKING TO YOUTH ABOUT SUBSTANCE USE

It's tricky. The dominant message to young people has always been abstinence only, like Just Say No and DARE (drug abuse resistance education) programs. But when you tell kids to just avoid it without discussing much else, you're only making them more curious about the substances. Kids need to explore their assumptions and beliefs—and ask questions.

Brandon and Celeste, parents who have navigated this discussion with their teens, shared what made their conversations effective. Here's what they had to say:

- They have made substance use a normal topic of discussion, rather than having pointed talks with their kids out of the blue.
- They've told their children that substance-use disorder runs in the family, and that may mean that their desire to use in the future could lead to larger consequences for them than for their friends. "We have the genetic predisposition to have issues with substances given our family history, so we want you to be aware of what this means for you when you're considering use." Sometimes they've likened this predisposition to an allergy, to make it easier for their kids' young minds to grasp, explaining that it's like how some people can tolerate certain foods, for example, and other people can't.

- They have emphasized that abstinence is the only guaranteed way to avoid the ramifications of drug and alcohol use, but acknowledged that they also know what it means to be a young person in a society that regularly turns to substances for fun and relief. "It's about having a truthful, open conversation. We know that demanding abstinence does not work, so we want to empower our kids to make decisions with the best information," Celeste says.
- They've answered questions about alcohol, opioids, and cannabis honestly, telling their children that we never know exactly how a brain will react, especially with a legacy of problematic use in a family. "I know that I can't stop my kids from ever using drugs or alcohol. And I don't want to, quite frankly. Drugs and alcohol are really helpful when we need them to be. I've needed prescription pain meds for my back and knee surgeries. They do the things we need them to do. I just want my kids to have as much information as possible so they feel empowered to make decisions," Brandon says.

We recommend taking a page out of Brandon and Celeste's book. Early on, talk to kids about substances:

- If you are having an alcoholic beverage, talk about what it is, and if they have any questions. Give space for kids to be curious without your judgment.
- Talk about how people use substances to change how they are feeling, and sometimes it becomes the only way they do this. Explore with your kids when they would know that substances are a problem and how they can come to you to talk about that at any time.
- Share any family stories of substance use issues and talk about what has happened. Truth and conversation are always better than secrets.
- Don't shy away from sharing your own relationship and experiences with substances. It can help kids understand what can go well and what might not.

HOW SUBSTANCE-USE DISORDER DEVELOPS

Substance use and mental health are intertwined. We've never worked with anybody who struggles with substances who didn't also struggle with self-worth, depression, anxiety, or difficulty in relationships. One condition does not cause another, but when we don't feel good about ourselves, substances can temporarily make us feel better. In the short term, it's an effective coping strategy—one that can become so reliable, it can supersede all others. But in the long-term, it can exacerbate existing mental health issues or even increase the risk of developing new ones.

Caitlyn was a competitive runner in high school, and although she didn't compete in college, she continued training. Like many at that age, she went through a bad relationship breakup and didn't have the emotional tools to cope with it. When she wasn't training hard for big goals, like qualifying for the Boston Marathon, she turned to alcohol. She also drank when she was injured and unable to run. "I had depression I wasn't dealing with," Caitlyn says. "So I coped with alcohol and running."

But when she was diagnosed in 2020 with dystonia, involuntary muscle contractions in the lower part of the body, running was no longer an option. She hit her bottom on July Fourth that year. Spending the day with friends and family, she was having problems walking. She drank a lot to cope, and by the time she got home, she was sobbing. "[My husband and I] were going to bed and I was really drunk," Caitlyn says. "I turned to him and told him I needed to go on antidepressants. I told him, 'I am having suicidal ideation.'"

By the time she woke up the next morning, Caitlyn's husband had already started researching treatment options. She started intense therapy and medication right away. She knew that she had to approach her recovery with an athlete's mind, she says, with the same dedication and commitment, going into a twelve-step program and also seeking support through Adult Children of Alcoholics. "With depression and certain events, I wish people would have recognized how much I was struggling. I don't think people knew how bad it really was," Caitlyn says. "Toward the last few months before I decided to stop, I was consciously aware it was becoming a problem again and I didn't care because I didn't want to have to deal with my stuff without it. I was ignoring the voice telling me to not go to the wine bar again today. I couldn't run and I didn't have this other way to deal with my unresolved stuff."

Although substance-use disorders usually begin with a conscious decision to use a substance, changes that occur in the brain at some point can turn casual use into a chronic, relapsing illness. Some people are predisposed to addiction almost immediately—the time is shorter between deciding to consume and becoming dependent on it to deal with life's hardships. The long-standing stigma is that everybody should know better, especially athletes. Shouldn't they, of all people, know how to make healthier decisions? But substance-use disorder doesn't develop in the prefrontal cortex, the part of the brain responsible for reasoning, problem-solving, and impulse control. Substance-use disorders actually manifest in the midbrain, where the pleasure center resides—the same place that tells us to eat food to survive and have sex to make a baby.

Stress also plays a role. And athletes, like everybody else, experience their share of stress, which can make it difficult to feel like good things are happening, even when they are. If an athlete feels overwhelmed by an upcoming competition, they will probably miss celebrating an academic achievement, for example. Stress is powerful, and when somebody is in a constant state of stress, the brain has a hard time registering anything positive. If you're already in a place of malaise, you may be more likely to use a substance to feel different.

Here's what happens, according to Kevin McCauley, MD, a naval flight surgeon for the Marine Corps heavy-lift helicopter and fighter/attack squadrons, who has studied the science of substance use[9]:

- When a person uses a substance, the midbrain releases dopamine, a powerful neurotransmitter, commonly known as the "feel-good" hormone.
- Since the feel-good feelings have been scarce (anhedonia), the neurotransmitters in the brain have been on empty and the alcohol or drug use adds fuel to the tank. This can feel like rocket fuel. (And who doesn't want to feel that good again and again and again?)
- Even though the prefrontal cortex may not agree (it's also in charge of judgment), the midbrain tells the prefrontal cortex that the substance is vital and imperative. The prefrontal cortex gets the message and reinforces to the midbrain that the substance is imperative.
- Then, when a stored cue (a psychological trigger, like a life stressor, the sight of the liquor store, or the sound of a wine bottle opening), is presented, the amygdala (the part of the brain that processes emotional responses) attaches a powerful emotional connection to the memory, the midbrain releases dopamine, and the prefrontal cortex tells the midbrain, again, that the substance is imperative.
- Due to this repetitive process, the brain is then rewired and the person loses the choice to control the use of the drug or alcohol.

When somebody is struggling with SUD, they may ask: why me? In families it's often hard to understand how substance use has had a significant impact on some members and not others, despite similar stressors and use. In Tiffany's family, for example, we see a history of severe substance use in various generations, but we can't screen or conduct genetic tests to find out who will fall to its power and who won't. All a person can do is identify factors that can heighten risk, like trauma, stress, or isolation, and develop effective coping strategies. The stress of sports, for example, presents another set of risk factors that may lead to substance use, but access to resources and a sense of connection can also alleviate them. Even these measures aren't guaranteed, though. Nothing related to substance-use disorder is formulaic.

What we do know, however, is that families and the systems that a person returns to after treatment for a substance-use disorder are important. If somebody puts the time and work in to make changes, but goes right back into a dynamic that is exactly the same as before, that person will likely revert back to the same coping mechanisms. A cornerstone of the twelve-step program is that a person needs to see change in their "people, places, and things" because the triggers are real and sometimes even deadly. When a person uses again, it's not because she's failed; it's because many factors contribute to it. It's important to suspend shame and blame—instead, offer support and turn toward what the person may need moving forward.

RULES, POLICIES, LAWS, AND ANTI-DOPING

Nearly all female athletes from college to the professional level are subject to the rules of organizations like the NCAA, the United States Anti-Doping Agency (USADA), and the World Anti-Doping Agency (WADA), which maintain lists of prohibited substances that either have the potential to enhance sport performance or pose a health risk to athletes. Those who are in any organization's drug-testing pool are subject to random, unannounced drug tests both outside of competition and in competition.

The reasons why athletes may cave to the temptation of cheating through drug use is complex. Some may operate under systems and coaches that force it upon them. Others may feel desperate to reach a certain level to earn money from sponsors or race prizes. Still others may want to prolong an athletic career—they don't know who they are without it. Sometimes substances can help relieve pain, speed the body's recovery between hard training sessions, or help with sleep. The pressure and win-at-all-costs culture can also contribute to the decision to take these drugs despite the risk of getting caught.

Athletes are responsible for knowing what kinds of supplements and prescription drugs they are permitted to take and when. Some substances are allowed outside competition but not in competition, while others require the athlete to get a therapeutic use exemption if a drug that is otherwise banned is needed for medical reasons. And these rules can also supersede local laws. While marijuana is legal in many states in the United States, for example, it is prohibited by WADA in competition (and thus, also banned by USADA, which abides by the list issued by WADA—the NCAA has looser rules regarding marijuana).

Sprinter Sha'Carri Richardson dazzled the track and field world at the 2021 US Olympic Trials, winning the hundred meters and qualifying for the Tokyo Games, only to find out she was suspended for one month after testing positive for marijuana. She accepted that she had violated the rule, explaining that she had found out that her mother had died and she used the substance to cope. She missed her first Olympics, where she likely would have contended for a medal, as a result (in fact, she went on to win the hundred-meter world championships in 2023). "I was definitely triggered and blinded by emotions, blinded by badness, and hurting, and hiding my hurt," Sha'Carri said during a *Today Show* interview. "I know I can't hide myself, so in some type of way, I was trying to hide my pain."

The controversy boiled over in the aftermath. Although almost a hundred other athletes in the past ten years have served suspensions for the same reason in the United States, it was Sha'Carri's case that caught fire. Some, including Sha'Carri, correctly pointed out that Black people are disproportionately punished in the United States for marijuana offenses. Others pointed out that the substance doesn't give a sprinter any advantage in competition; in fact, it might hinder it. Nonetheless, Travis Tygart, CEO of USADA, said that the agency was bound by WADA policy. "This is true even in sad and tough cases like this one, where we might take a different approach if the choice was ours to make," he said, adding, "the real issue here is trying to find ways to support athletes who find themselves dealing with mental health issues similar to [Sha'Carri]."

Today, more athletes are speaking out about their use of cannabis for other reasons, including pain management. WNBA sensation Brittney

Griner may be the most prominent, after she was detained in Russia in 2022 when customs officials found vape cartridges containing hashish oil, which is illegal in Russia, in her luggage. Her lawyers said that Brittney had been authorized to use medicinal cannabis in her home state of Arizona, where she plays for the Phoenix Mercury, though it is banned in the WNBA. Brittney and other WNBA players compete in other countries in the offseason to make more money (NBA players make forty-four times what the average WNBA athlete makes), and no doubt, Brittney has endured her share of injuries that require some kind of relief.

Opioids can pose a particular risk to athletes who often have to undergo surgeries for various injuries. They either have to experience a lot of pain during recovery or risk dependency on these highly addictive substances. The Delaware Department of Health and Social Services and the Department of Services for Children, Youth and Their Families are collaborating on a project aimed to prevent opioid[10] use among young athletes by funding educational programs in the community, including a youth football team, basketball league, and a lacrosse team. The program also aims to help young players and their parents learn how to cope with stress, as well as healthy ways to manage nutrition and sleep. The preventative approach is hopefully lowering the risk for substance-use disorder while teaching athletes how to deal with injuries, pressure to perform, and anxiety without using substances.

We know that prevention is always better than treatment and that successful prevention is an ongoing endeavor. Caitlyn, for one, says she wakes up every day and makes a conscious decision not to drink. She channels the mental focus she once used to run marathons to help her stay on track and uncover her self-worth outside of sport. "If you have any inkling within yourself that you are struggling, listen to it," she says. "My whole identity was wrapped up in running and now I'm on a lifelong journey of unwrapping that—it can perpetuate substance [use]. Get curious who you are outside your sport . . . you are more than that."

Chapter Eleven

THE PARADOX OF SOCIAL MEDIA

Athletes are vulnerable to the same mental health
pitfalls of social media as everybody else, but female
athletes can also leverage it for good.

So many teenage athletes feel a constant obligation to their phones, posting their daily highlight reels, choosing their most flattering angles, and smiling for their selfies each day—even on the days that they don't feel as happy as they appear. A sixteen-year-old elite gymnast told us how she feels like she has to be "on" at all times. She's waiting for calls from top coaches at coveted NCAA programs—and she's well aware that those coaches are probably already getting to know her from afar via Instagram or TikTok or anywhere her digital presence exists. "I feel like I have to post everything I'm doing to show how well-rounded I am during the recruiting process," she says. "I don't want to be 'just an athlete.' I want to document that I'm a strong student and I volunteer, too." She's bright, motivated, engaging—and utterly preoccupied with her appearance. "I never get a break. Everybody knows my every move," the gymnast says.

Like nearly all young people, this gymnast feels pressure to show that they're out and about, whether that means posting videos and photos of their social activities or "checking in" to their location so everybody can see what they're up to (and that they haven't been excluded). Nobody wants to feel uninvited, left out, or like a bore for checking in at home instead of meeting up with friends. She wants to feel included in all the activities she knows her teammates and friends will attend but also has a deep desire to just "go off the grid" because she realizes she needs a break.

Striving for perfection is hard enough. Creating a mirage of perfection online is exhausting. It leaves the teen athlete feeling depleted. And the gymnast we spoke with is far from alone—according to the Pew Research Center, 92 percent of tweens and teenagers are active on social media, and girls spend more than two hours each day on it, beginning around age eleven. At a key juncture in their development, when adolescent brains are still growing and young people are starting to figure out their identity, they're turning to a constant feed of idealized versions of what they think their lives—and their bodies—should look like. They compare themselves to filtered or carefully selected photos of peers or celebrities (or their favorite athletes), and they begin to measure their popularity and self-worth in followers and likes.

While all that sounds really bad, we also have to understand that the kinds of connection and socialization older generations forged in real life now happen digitally. If you're wondering why your teen is "always" on her phone, it's likely because she doesn't want to miss out on the inside joke, the funny meme, or what her friends are gossiping about after school. That sense of connection isn't inherently bad. Young people are more attuned to current events, causes, and activism because of social media, and they can find a sense of belonging regarding gender or sexual identity, too. They find new interests and hobbies because they're exposed to such a wide variety of information. They can connect with and draw inspiration from other athletes in their sport pretty much anywhere in the world. These are all great reasons to allow kids to explore online.

Social media can become problematic, however, when it infringes on sleep, provokes anxiety or depression, leads to bullying and trolling, or encourages disordered eating, all of which can easily happen, especially for girls and young women, according to a growing body of research. It behooves parents and caregivers to help their daughters learn how to have a healthy relationship with social media and have frequent conversations with them about it. Just like substances, forbidding its use will not work. It's not going anywhere, and as they advance in their athletic careers, at least in this era, social media will continue to play a part in their experiences. While it can have an extremely positive influence at times, inevitably, she will also encounter her share of negativity, especially if she goes on to compete in college or professionally, putting her more in the public eye. Helping her discover the role she'd like social media to have in her life is essential, as well as teaching her to notice signs that it's time to reevaluate her relationship with it.

For older generations, it's always going to be difficult to keep up with which platforms their kids are using and how they interact with people online. It's constantly changing and evolving. Today, it's Snapchat, TikTok, and Instagram. Tomorrow, it may be Roblox, Discord, and BeReal. The next day, it will be something we've never heard of. The basic principles remain the same, though: you want your young athlete to know exactly why she's using it. Ask her periodically how she feels after an hour scrolling on her phone, but be careful not to approach social media use with judgment—as we've suggested so many times throughout this book, express curiosity by asking open-ended questions about what your teen is seeing and experiencing. Let them teach you about the newest platforms they're on and what they like and don't like about them. With the right blend of curiosity, along with setting limits and boundaries appropriately and in line with your family values, social media can remain an asset for young people.

For example, Suzy Rosen, a licensed therapist in Bend, Oregon, who specializes in working with teens and their families, has talked to many young people who say they feel relieved when their parents put their phones away for them. While they may resist boundaries, roll their eyes, or even get angry at times, they often discover that when their phones are stored outside of their bedrooms, they sleep better, or when they take a break from screens during dinner, they feel rejuvenated. Giving them a chance to realize that now will help them form healthier habits as they grow up. "The most important thing to remember is that teenagers were basically born with these phones in their hands and they were not given a choice," Rosen says. "Back in the day, if you did something stupid, three people saw it and it stopped there. Today it goes however far their reach is on social media."

CONNECTIONS AND COMPARISONS

For Rose, the high school basketball player in the Pacific Northwest, social media "feels like pressure," she says. The photos that are posted to the team's platforms are sometimes a source of embarrassment; they aren't the pictures she would have chosen. For example, she remembers a shot of herself mid layup, which was a game-changing move and should have been a source of pride. "But I had a horrendous game face on, so I was not going to show that accomplishment on social media," Rose says.

Her friend Camille, a runner, agrees. She's only ever posted photos of herself holding a trophy or after she's crossed the finish line; rarely does she show herself actually running. "Running pictures have to be so particular," she says, explaining that her leg muscles have to look good and her face has to have the right expression, too. Rose says that for female athletes to get a bigger following, they have to be attractive. "A lot of athletes who are equally as good as the pretty girls don't get the same attention online," she says. "It's like, 'Oh my gosh, she has it all because she is good *and* pretty.'"

While sports are inclusive of so many body types, from powerlifters to throwers to sprinters to gymnasts, one of the biggest risks for girls and women using apps like Instagram and TikTok remains falling into the comparison traps and negative body image, which can lead to problems like depression, anxiety, and eating disorders. One area of concern

171

for young female athletes is comparing their bodies not only with each other but also with the older professional athletes they follow. We have to remind girls that the women they look up to haven't always looked the way they do now—and that athletes compete their best with all different body types, and our healthy bodies change many times throughout our lives.

Jessica and Justin are raising two teen daughters and know that conversations about social media use are ongoing. They do see some value in it, however. Their daughter MacKenzie was able to see herself in the bodies of water polo players she spied online after Justin pointed them out and was instantly interested in the sport. "It was the women's Olympic team, and almost all the players had power thighs and shoulders and were over six feet tall," Justin says. "MacKenzie was like, 'Oh my gosh, they look exactly like me!' and I think it was so huge for her to feel like she's an athlete."

But it's not just photos of pro athletes that girls are exposed to. They also see and may also try to mimic what pros eat or drink. Again, it's important to emphasize that fueling and nutrition are different for an adult athlete versus somebody who's still growing. Even when they become fully grown, nutritional needs and preferences are still highly individual. It's great to pick up a new recipe for something that looks delicious, but it's not beneficial to copy anybody else's "what I eat in a day" reel. Following superstar athletes is a wonderful avenue for learning how they train, how they take care of themselves, and what they do outside of sport, for example, but teens should understand that the intensity and volume of training is something they've worked toward over many years, and they shouldn't try to replicate it as adolescents.

One of the most publicized examples of how social media can be damaging for young people came from a lawsuit against Meta (the company that owns Facebook and Instagram) in 2022, filed on behalf of Alexis Spence by the Social Media Victims Law Center,[1] an organization that advocates for families of teens who have been harmed online. As a preteen, the suit alleges, Alexis's "addictive" use of Instagram resulted in an eating disorder, self-harm, and suicidal thoughts. The lawsuit cites Meta's own research,[2] leaked to the media in 2022, showing that the company knew that its technology exacerbated body image and mental health issues among teenage girls. According to court documents, Alexis, at age eleven, started an Instagram account without her parents' knowledge (and in violation of the platform's minimum age of thirteen), and Instagram's artificial intelligence engine (the algorithm) relentlessly presented her content that glorified anorexia and self-harming, including videos and online groups that encouraged eating disorders. Six years later, Alexis is in recovery after hospitalizations for depression, anxiety, and anorexia (the case was still underway in fall 2023).

Alexis's story also highlights why adolescents are particularly vulnerable to the addictive nature of social media. They're going through the second-biggest period of brain growth—and the part of the brain that is involved in decision-making isn't fully developed until age twenty-five. According to several studies and behavioral health experts, that means that teenagers are rewiring their brains to seek out immediate gratification—shares, likes, and comments—that trigger the reward center, which drives surges of dopamine. The result is addiction, similar to using substances or gambling, which is why overusing these apps can result in so many mental health issues.

It's helpful to continue asking young athletes what they're getting out of the time they're spending on Instagram, TikTok, or other apps and what their intentions are in using the apps. Some of the questions that may elicit further dialogue include: How are you feeling after you've been looking at social media today? What did you see that activated unusual or uncomfortable emotions? How do you feel differently about yourself now versus before you looked at your accounts today? Regular and frequent conversations will help you flag potential trouble spots and will help your athlete process her online experience. Think of it this way: if your daughter had her teammates over for pizza, you'd likely observe their interactions and hear what they're talking about.

That's always been the case for parents and caregivers and has always served as a way to monitor behavior and gather intelligence about what might be going on in their lives, as well as what they're listening to and watching. It just takes a bit more effort to get that information now because it isn't happening around your kitchen table as often anymore. Talking with girls about what they are engaging with on social media, expressing trust, and encouraging open dialogue will help you both navigate this world without a constant need to monitor their feeds.

BEWARE THE BULLY

Ally, a member of the acrobatics and tumbling team at a private university on the east coast, still has an up-and-down relationship with social media. In her sport, competitors keep a close eye on each other's accounts and spend a lot of time comparing themselves. She's watched teammates block each other on apps or post unflattering stories about team members when they aren't getting along.

Bullying comes in many different forms on the web. Some of it comes from classmates or teammates, like in Ally's case. Other times, it comes from strangers (let's call them trolls) or people who follow the sport (we'd like to call them fans, but if they're publicly ridiculing the athletes they follow, they don't deserve that title). With the rise in legalized gambling, including in college sports, bettors are now also abusing and threatening athletes who they blame for losing a game on which they had placed money. It's all to say that, once upon a time, players could make a mistake in a game and feel a little miserable and embarrassed about it, but at least few people beyond the confines of the playing field would know about it. Now, of course, everybody has a camera and everybody has an Instagram account, so that mistake goes viral. People in the far corners of the world can now know that Joselyn, the left fielder from the Anytown High School softball team, fell flat on her face while running to catch a fly ball, and it was hilarious. Just imagine fifteen-year-old Joselyn coping with an endless scroll of teasing and taunts from her bedroom in Anytown, which she vows to never leave again. While it may seem far-fetched, it happens often enough that the mere threat or fear of it can be a source of anxiety.

When we talk about the problem of perfectionism, which can result in severe anxiety among young female athletes, it isn't just emanating from insecurity. It's also a survival tactic. So many are afraid to make mistakes because they don't want to become the next Joselyn. Having high expectations is admirable, of course, but when people develop a crippling fear of failure, kids (and adults, for that matter) stop learning and growing. They won't try to master new skills or interests, preferring to stick with what they know they're already good at. Perfectionism also leads to burnout: it's exhausting to keep up a flawless record.

The 2021 Tokyo Olympics offered its share of case studies, most notably when Simone Biles, the most decorated gymnast in US history, withdrew from competition. She set a great example for younger athletes who may hesitate to ever take a mental health break, saying she knew that if she pressed forward, she would likely injure herself while competing and may even cost the team a medal. "We have to protect our body and our mind," she said during a press conference in Tokyo, later reminding fans, "we're not just athletes; we're people at the end of the day." While many fans cheered her decision and flooded social media with messages of support, Simone also faced bullying, racism, and backlash from the most ignorant people on social media, talk radio, and the like. We won't rehash exact statements here, but we will applaud Simone for how she prioritized her well-being, despite this cruelty. It wasn't, after all, the first time she'd encountered bullying. Growing up, she was made fun of at school for her muscular build, developed through hard work at the gym. And in 2016, she was attacked on Instagram for her physique and appearance as well. Biles responded: "You all can judge my body all you want, but at the end of the day it's MY body. I love it & I'm comfortable in my skin."[3]

Serena Williams, widely referred to as the world's all-time best tennis player, has not been exempt from online attacks and body-shaming, even from the mainstream media. Sadly, the examples are numerous, but one 2015 *New York Times* article that focused on female players' appearances and body types[4] set off a firestorm of backlash on social media. Kareem Abdul-Jabbar even wrote a piece in *Time* magazine[5] about it, calling it a "racist rejection of Black women's bodies that don't conform to the traditional body shapes of white athletes and dancers."

After the 2021 Summer Games, a study conducted by World Athletics,[6] the governing body of international track and field, confirmed what many already assumed: female athletes received 87 percent of all targeted online abuse during the Olympics. The research used a sample of 161 Twitter handles of athletes involved in Tokyo, tracking the accounts beginning one week before the opening ceremony and concluding the day after the closing ceremony. It found sexist, racist, transphobic, and homophobic abuse of the athletes, as well as unfounded doping accusations. World Athletics conducted a similar study during the 2022 World Championships,[7] which were held in Eugene, Oregon, and this time included Instagram accounts of 461 athletes. The results showed that 60 percent of detected online abuse was sexual or racial (including use of the N-word and monkey emojis). Again, the targets of the attacks were mostly women.

Holly Bradshaw, a British pole-vaulter who won the bronze medal in Tokyo, came forward[8] when the World Athletics studies were released to share her account of bullying and harassment during the 2022 World Championships, where she had to withdraw from competition after her pole broke during a warm-up vault and she injured herself. Some trolls blamed the mishap on her weight and others accused her of attention-seeking, saying she was just being "weak."

Of course, it wasn't the first time Bradshaw had encountered social media abuse: she had long been criticized for her appearance, since the 2012 Olympics. "It was kind of coming at me from all different angles. I was like, 'What if I am fat? I am overweight?' Then, I spent a year when I would skip meals. I would drastically cut portion sizes because if this is what people are saying about me, I need to lose weight,"

Bradshaw told Olympics.com. The experiences have led her to strategize better about what she reads and when. "I'll definitely have a social media block for a week or two weeks before a major championship, and I don't want to do it, but if I'm the day out from the Olympic final and someone posts a comment as negative . . . that upsets my mindset."

The bullying, body-shaming, and abuse that can happen on every platform are valid reasons why athletes might choose to use them in moderation. Teaching young athletes how to insulate themselves from attacks will help them navigate these issues later.

FORMING HEALTHY SOCIAL MEDIA PRACTICES

Athletes can benefit from social media, no doubt—building connections, learning skills, and even making some money. But forming a healthy relationship with social media is a life skill. Otherwise, it can become addictive and have detrimental effects on mental health. Here are a few tips to help young women and girls make sure that their social media use remains positive:

1. **Take inventory of who you're following.** How do the people, brands, and groups you are connected to make you feel? When you scroll through your timeline, it shouldn't leave you feeling sad, depressed, overwhelmed, anxious, or jealous. If certain accounts make your self-esteem plummet, then unfollow them. If somebody is consistently rude or negative, then block them. Your feed should make you feel good—motivated, happy, inspired, and curious.

2. **Think about what you share and how you comment.** Young people, especially, don't often think of the long-term impact of what they say or do online. It's forever, so think carefully before you post or comment. What is the purpose of the post? What are you trying to accomplish by it? And are your comments helpful or

hurtful to others? When you feel the urge to disparage or disagree with others on social media more often than you're compelled to post encouragement or connection, it might be time to take a break from it.

3. **Set limits.** Your phone is always nearby, and it's easy to constantly check Instagram or TikTok whenever you're bored, but your mind needs time to do nothing. When you carve out space in your day to daydream or just have uninterrupted moments with others, you think more clearly, sleep more soundly, and focus more easily.

4. **Take periodic breaks.** Always set aside a day, week, or longer to log off from the noise. It gives you the chance to evaluate if you're spending too much time on social media, if it's making you feel anxious, depressed, or otherwise bad about yourself, and if it is taking away time you could spend with teammates, friends, or family. When you eliminate it from your routine for a period of time, it's healthy and eye-opening to see what kind of influence it has in your life.

PLATFORMS WITH PURPOSE

Of course, up until social media became widely used, female athletes had to rely on paltry mainstream media coverage to gain any coverage of their stories. As players have told their own stories on their own platforms, their sports have only grown in popularity, especially at the Olympic and professional level. Even at the high school level, girls understand the power of their smartphones to drum up support for their big competitions; they often don't feel that school administrators will do it for them. "You have to be a marketer if you are a female athlete," Rose says.

The WNBA is a primary example of how an entire league and its individual players have leveraged their social media presence not only to increase viewership and fan base but to also rally around causes that are important to them. The Atlanta Dream, for example, endorsed Rev. Raphael Warnock's campaign for the 2020 Georgia Senate race, wore

Black Lives Matter shirts at games (a movement that Warnock's opponent, who was co-owner of their team at the time, did not support), and posted the images on their channels. The league also joined forces on social media to push for star Brittney Griner's release from imprisonment in Russia in 2022, using the #WeAreBG hashtag (as we mentioned in chapter 9, she was in Russia to play in the offseason to earn extra money but was detained at an airport for carrying a small amount of marijuana concentrate in her luggage. She was released after ten months).

And who could forget when Sedona Prince, then a member of the women's basketball team at the University of Oregon, leveraged her TikTok[9] following to draw attention to the huge disparities between the facilities and financial support allotted to the men's and women's 2021 NCAA tournaments? She showed a single rack of dumbbells the women were given, compared to a fully outfitted gym that the men had access to, along with other examples showing the difference between the meals and swag that the women received compared to the men. The video stoked outrage on the internet and launched a full-fledged investigation into equity of the NCAA's broadcast and corporate contracts, revenue distribution, organizational structure, and culture. According to a 114-page report by the law firm of civil rights attorney Roberta A. Kaplan,[10] the NCAA "normalized" and perpetuated gender inequities—a fact that Prince's TikTok campaign helped bring to light.

By 2023, the women's NCAA Final Four tournament was shattering viewership records. The championship game between Louisiana State and Iowa drew 9.9 million viewers, making it, at the time, the most viewed college sporting event ever on ESPN+.[11] Fans, new and old, were enthralled by the rivalry between two star players, Angel Reese of LSU, and Caitlin Clark from Iowa. Now, the NCAA estimates that the women's tournament could be worth $85 million by 2025 compared to the $6 million 2023 agreement with ESPN.[12] Recall that this growth began because of a player's TikTok video that led to the needed scrutiny of equity in the NCAA.

This is what we mean by having a purpose for social media use—it can play an important role in defining values and pushing for change when athletes give it a clear role in their lives. While mainstream media still gives far less attention to women's sports in comparison to men's, female athletes have made direct connections with their fans, grown interest, and drawn far more attention not only to their sports but also their causes by building their followings online. It's become far more effective to build an audience on Instagram (for example) than via television or newspapers.

WHAT A WAY TO MAKE A LIVING

College athletes now have the opportunity to monetize their social media followings through "Name, Image, and Likeness" (NIL) deals—and high school athletes in many states are also gaining permission to capitalize on the same kinds of sponsorships. We're not going to lie. Understanding NIL in 2024 is a challenge: the rules and oversight are constantly changing and, full disclosure, it might all look very different in the months and years to come. The basic idea, however, is that athletes can now earn money and build their brands while competing in sports. It used to be illegal for student athletes to receive compensation outside of scholarships. But in July 2021, the US Supreme Court ruled that the NCAA couldn't limit education-related payments to athletes, allowing states to determine new NIL rules, and in the absence of state policy, colleges and universities could decide. Now a large number of student athletes can sign endorsements, profit from corporate sponsorships, and get paid to coach or appear at fan events, sign autographs, and more.

This change in policy has been a game changer for many female athletes. Angel Reese, the LSU basketball star, for example, said she will likely opt to remain in the NCAA for the remainder of her eligibility because it's become more lucrative than what her salary would probably be as a pro in the WNBA. On3, an NIL sports media platform, estimated Reese's earnings as a sophomore at $1.3 million per year.[13] In 2022, the average WNBA salary was $102,751.[14]

As a steeplechaser at Duke University, Emily Cole has also made out well in her NIL pursuit, bringing in an estimated $144,000[15] in 2023 through partnerships with Dicks Sporting Goods, Garmin, Champs Sports, and others, as well as publishing her book *The Players' Plate: An Unorthodox Guide to Sport Nutrition.* As of fall 2023, she had 183,000 followers on Instagram and 316,000 on TikTok, making her platform an attractive draw for many brands to pedal their products.

The book was a direct outcome of a health crisis Cole suffered during her high school years in Texas. It was then that she began doing a lot of cooking for herself in an effort to "eat healthy" and drinking as much water as she could, assuming she needed a lot of fluid while training in the Houston heat. Just before her state cross-country meet her senior year, she slipped into a coma as a result of hyponatremia, a condition when the sodium level in your blood is too low and the fluid in the body is high; water moves into body cells, causing brain tissues to swell. After Cole recovered, writing *The Player's Plate* became a way to process what had happened and also help other athletes better understand their nutritional and fueling needs.

The book helped launch Cole as an NIL trailblazer and clarify her mission to help others have a healthy relationship with food. She's careful about which companies she works with and has an audience that shares her passion. But Cole understands that brand promotion is also an extra full-time job, on top of many hours of training, classes, studying, traveling, and socializing. It's not for everybody and can easily overwhelm younger athletes, she says. "Social media and NIL are something to be wary of if you don't have a defined objective," she says. "It can be detrimental to mental health, and it's another thing that needs to be done when it's your job—you have to create content. Some athletes stay up late, working to create, and then it impacts their sleep and productivity."

Many of these NIL partnerships also require athletes to post more frequently than they otherwise would, which means more time spent on their phones. A growing body of research by Leornaro S. Fortes, a sport and exercise neuroscientist at the Federal University of Paraiba, Brazil,[16] suggests that repeated social media use on smartphones immediately before training sessions may reduce or nullify training gains and endurance performance. Caroline Doty, the former assistant coach of the women's basketball team at the University of Wisconsin, saw the direct effects of social media use combined with NIL responsibilities. "The athletes have to travel to do video shoots and that can take away from team bonding, for example," she says. "When I was an athlete, the focus was basketball. We created our own bubble and there wasn't a lot of outside noise. Now there are so many distractions."

But for Cole, NIL has been nothing but a positive and life-changing experience. It's allowed her to generate more awareness for her sport and elevate the women who are part of it, which allows those sports to grow in a way they never have. And that's been the key for many other athletes across the country, too. Although football earns more than half of all the money flowing into NIL deals, at the end of 2022, women's basketball ranked third among NIL-compensated sports, earning 12.6 percent of the pie, according to Opendorse,[17] one of the online platforms where athletes strike NIL deals (men's basketball was second, with 19 percent of earnings). In fact, six women's sports were in the top ten for NIL sports—women's basketball, volleyball, and softball (which even beat baseball in these rankings).

NIL allows women to earn a living from sports in a way that they never have before; they don't currently have a shot at the salaries male athletes make in the NBA or NFL, so capitalizing on the opportunities while they exist can set them up for long-term success. Unfortunately, however, the system is, as always, rewarding white athletes whose images (and stereotypical white beauty) are deemed more appealing to audiences, leaving a lot of athletes of color without access to the same chances to profit off their talent. And many young people don't have the financial literacy to manage the money they're making, either—few people are guiding their decisions or teaching them how to invest or save it.

Angelina, the distance running coach at Ball State University in Indiana, cautions that although the upsides of increased income for athletes is attractive, it has some downsides, too. "Some kids are making nothing," she says, adding that their experience of who companies want to have as the face of their organizations and in the Midwest exposes athletes of color to lot of racism. Moreover, she says that expressions and gestures during the heat of competition are interpreted differently depending on the color of the athlete's skin—and Black athletes, for example, feel compelled to spend a lot of money on hair braiding to look "acceptable" for photo shoots and team picture days due to the blatant racism. "My darker skin Black girls feel like they are not as pretty as their lighter skin teammates and the [lighter skinned athletes] get better sponsorship packages and NIL deals. It has nothing to do with how good they are athletically, but rather how they look."

Livvy Dunne, an All-America gymnast at Louisiana State, was the highest-ranking female NIL athlete in 2023, earning an estimated $3.5 million in 2023,[18] with more than nine million social media followers. She's partnered with brands like Vuori Clothing and American Eagle. Her massive following has been lucrative, but not without a cost. After hundreds of teenage boys surrounded the team bus to get a glimpse of Livvy at a 2023 competition against the University of Utah in Salt Lake City, the police had to escort athletes from both teams to exit the facility safely. It's just one of many repercussions that officials never considered when NIL went into effect—and as an aside, it was Livvy who received the backlash after the Utah incident, with onlookers saying she "brought it on herself" by having such a large online presence.

NIL will continue to be a tricky area for athletes. When one player gets a deal that another player wants, it only creates more competition among teammates and amplifies the pressures they're facing. Will they play through injuries to satisfy the terms of a contract? Will they say or do something that might jeopardize a deal? The added responsibilities of photo shoots, appearances, and creating massive amounts of content take a lot of time away from recovery and sleep. When athletes get stressed, overwhelmed, and don't get enough rest, they suffer. Because the rules and landscape are constantly changing when it comes to NIL, we have a lot to learn along the way. At this point, we recommend a slow approach that allows an athlete to monitor not just their earnings but also how it impacts their emotions and time commitments. Conversations about costs and benefits are always valuable.

Chapter Twelve

NAVIGATING OUR BODIES
AND OUR CHOICES

Female athletes have a lot to manage when it comes to
physical health and reproductive function. Getting help,
support, and information remains challenging.

It was an awkward and confusing situation to find herself in as a young
college athlete. A volleyball player on the East Coast, competing for a
Division III program, had always looked up to her teammate, who was
two years older, as a leader and a trusted source of support to the new-
comers on the team. But one day their roles abruptly reversed. Cut off
from her parents and with no access to transportation, the older player
needed a ride to the pharmacy to buy a pregnancy test. So the younger
teammate (who preferred not to be named here) stepped up in a way
that required a lot of maturity from a nineteen-year-old.

The pregnancy test confirmed what the older player had suspected.
Now she needed more than just a ride to the drug store. She needed a
best friend, somebody who would hold her hand, literally and figura-
tively, through appointments and difficult conversations in the following weeks. "I took her to a doctor to get blood tests and stuff," the
younger player says. "We didn't really know what to do." Eventually

they went to their coach, who was somebody they described as compassionate and empathetic—a mom herself. She connected the player, who wanted to continue her pregnancy, with the medical resources she needed, and with the athlete's permission, the coach asked doctors if it was safe for the defensive specialist (a position that demands a lot of saves, digs, and physicality) to continue training. But between the pregnancy and the onset of the COVID-19 pandemic, the athlete decided to leave the university. Even with that key support in place, she did not return to campus to finish her degree. According to the National Center for Education Statistics, parents are ten times less likely to complete a bachelor's degree within five years than peers without children.

Leslie Lu, another Division III volleyball player at a mid-Atlantic university, also went through what she called a "pregnancy scare." She too wasn't sure what to do, so she went to the campus health center, where they gave her a pregnancy test and screened for sexually transmitted infections. As an athlete on the small, close-knit campus, Leslie Lu wasn't sure who to trust or talk to about her options, so she decided to handle it alone. "I wish everyone in our community would be more comfortable talking about reproductive health in general," she says.

These athletes' experiences are not unique. We asked a lot of women from a variety of sports, geographic regions, and NCAA divisions how their coaches and athletic departments approach women's health. After all, their performances and educational opportunities are directly linked to how well their bodies function. But with barely an exception, the athletes responded that it was rarely or never talked about. The lack of guidance can quickly become devastating for athletes at a time when bodily autonomy and private health care choices are under direct political attack in the United States, stripping women, transgender, and nonbinary people in large swaths of the country of the right to decide when to have a family or receive gender-affirming care. We know that the ability to control when and if we have a child is linked to socioeconomic standing: as the American Psychological Association and other experts point out, the laws restricting access to safe and legal abortions are most likely to affect people of color, sexual and gender identity minorities, as well as those who reside in medically underserved regions. Adding barriers to reproductive health services increases stress, anxiety, and depression. The diminishing rights to abortion and the denial of gender-affirming treatments are interconnected and coordinated—they take away our freedom to decide who we are and what we want our futures to look like. And these policies target people who are already marginalized.

Nonetheless, the closest thing to reproductive health discussion that the athletes told us they consistently received was an annual Title IX policy information session, as the law pertains to sexual harassment, sexual violence, and coercion. "They show us this cheesy 'consent' video at the beginning of the school year, but that's about it," an athlete in one of our collegiate focus groups says, as the rest of the cohort nodded in agreement.

While we applaud the education on important issues related to Title IX, it does not begin to touch the surface of what female athletes need to know to train and perform their best. Understanding their hormonal fluctuations, periods, and options related to birth control, pregnancy, postpartum health, and fertility is paramount to improving mental health. All of these factors are heavy burdens for girls and women to carry on their own. Making all of these topics less taboo would go a long way toward alleviating fear, anxiety, and confusion—and it would free up a lot of headspace that could be devoted to improving skills and competition.

The athletes we spoke with took a guess that many male coaches, in particular, shy away from talking about women's reproductive health because it seems like a sexualized and uncomfortable conversation. Coaches might lack the training or education they need to approach these topics appropriately and with confidence. And in many cases, the athletes who have played for male and female coaches acknowledge that women are much more adept at normalizing open dialogue about women's health. "When I have one-on-one conversations with the athletes, I'll straight-up ask them if they're having a period, and I do not believe that if I was a male coach that I would be able to have that conversation," says Brooke, a head cross-country coach at a mid-Atlantic university. "I want male coaches to have that power—where they're able to ask and not have it come off in the wrong way. Because your period affects your training and what's happening to your body."

We fully support and advocate for recruiting and retaining more female coaches across all sports, but we also believe that with encouragement and training, men are able and (most often) willing to learn how to talk about this part of their athletes' health. It's basic biology, a science-based discussion that alleviates athlete misconceptions and general unease about their bodies and the options they have related to their reproductive function. That said, the issue of women's health is a hot potato of sorts: whose responsibility is it to provide information, guidance, and care? Coaches are often the go-to, catch-all for everything, but they shouldn't (and can't) be. They, along with athletic trainers, can be a referral resource to health care providers—but learning how to navigate the basics of what their athletes feel and experience every day, as well as understanding the choices they need to make about their bodies, should be everybody's role.

PERIODS AND PERFORMANCE

While we've already covered how periods can influence a girls' participation in sports during puberty, we also know that menstruation has a big impact on performance throughout an athletic career. Jen, an assistant coach at an NCAA Division I cross-country program in the Northeast, educates the women on her team about why their performances may not always match their expectations while they're still developing in college. Yes, women's development continues into the post–high school years, too—and a lot of people don't talk about that, which can leave female athletes demoralized on occasion. "If we start focusing on their athletic performance over their growth and development, then their growth and development don't happen," Jen says. "And that could be physiologically with their bones and muscles, but it also can affect their brain growth as well."

Reinforcing the conversations about the connection between low energy availability (LEA), bone health, reproductive health, and mental health is essential. Jen has given her athletes books to read about properly fueling their active lives and also keeps dialogue going throughout the year, trying to check in with how everybody is doing with casual conversations before practices and afterward. But joining the women's team during an easy run is where Jen says, "I get the real tea." Running together side by side, when nobody feels forced to have eye contact, allows the runners to more easily open up about the good, the bad, and everything in between. Jen believes the more they can talk about menstrual cycles and their effect on performance, the better the athletes can cope with the ups and downs. "At least if they know why they might be struggling sometimes, they're not beating themselves up over what feels like a lousy training session or if I know what's going on, we can adapt and change the workout, if that helps," she says. "It's really just having a conversation and not letting the coach's ego get in the way. If a runner comes to you and says a workout isn't working for them that day, be receptive to hearing how they feel."

Professional athletes are also trying to normalize the conversation and celebrate their periods as a vital sign—an indicator of their health, instead of something to dread or feel ashamed about. Emma Pallant-Browne, for example, three-time World Duathlon champion, responded to a photo of herself that circulated after a triathlon she raced in May 2023. If you look carefully, you can see blood stains on her race kit—and apparently some people looked *that* closely. Instead of feeling embarrassed, Emma used it as an opportunity to talk about menstruation as an athlete.

"If you wrote to me saying 99% of the women you know would have been mortified at this then that is exactly why I am sharing this, because there really is nothing wrong," she wrote on Instagram.[1] "It's natural, and coming from eating issues as an endurance runner when I was growing up where I didn't have my period, I now see it as beautiful. So if you have a photo like this, save it, cherish it, remember how you performed on a tough day because one day you might just be able to help someone else with it."

Research into how menstruation affects athletic performance is relatively new and still evolving. But coaches have more information now about when menstruating athletes could benefit from extra recovery, when they might be at more risk of injuries like ACL tears due to loosening ligaments and tendons, and at what point each month they might maximize strength training or endurance work (but, again, we are also individuals, and we haven't yet discovered any magic formulas for leveraging our hormonal fluctuations as superpowers). Such research provides more context about optimizing fueling and nutrition strategies and adaptations based on when hormone levels change. All of these stages of the cycle directly influence an athlete's mental health, too—research suggests that the physical discomfort of having a period can lead to decreased self-esteem, irritability, and contribute to depression.

Sade, the triathlete at a Division III Midwestern school, gives credit to her female coaches for including periods as a key factor in their expectations of the team. It sends a message that they don't have to hide what's going on and they can talk openly about how they feel. "One of us had a bad race and the coach asked, 'What happened? Normally that's not what your times look like. Is anything going on?' And my teammate just said, 'Yeah, I have my period,'" she says. "Our coach was like, 'Got it.' And that was the end of the conversation."

A BODY OF DECISIONS

Unfortunately, Elizabeth Carey, a long-time high school track and field coach in Seattle and a frequent speaker on reproductive health at coaches' conventions, as well as author of *Girls Running: All You Need to Strive, Thrive, and Run Your Best*, says she sees more hesitancy than ever in some areas of the country to discuss athlete reproductive health, including periods and birth control. Shame, fear, and politicization are getting in the way of science. "These cultural influences really affect the athlete's ability to deal with periods and birth control, because they're dealing with so many confounding pressures around it—each girl's journey is unique and dependent upon their family, their socioeconomic background, their location, and the politics around that," she says.

Allison, who played water polo for a Division I university in the mid-Atlantic, came from Canada to attend college and compete in the NCAA. Now she's working on her PhD, studying female athletes and reproductive health, focusing on their choices and how they make them. During her undergraduate studies, she took one women's health class and was struck by how little she knew about her own body and the options she had. It actually led her to change the contraception she was using at the time to a hormonal intrauterine device (IUD)—an option her doctor hadn't told her about. Prior to getting an IUD, she was taking Depo Provera, which required an injection every three months. Coming from Canada, where the universal health care system is publicly funded, she ran into problems in the United States trying to get her shot when she needed it. "I went to our team doctor and told her what birth control I was on. I had the prescription and everything—I just needed a doctor to inject it. And she couldn't do it because it wasn't covered under my insurance as an athlete," Allison says. "She told me I could come to her private practice for it, but it was forty-five minutes away from campus and I didn't have a car. If I had known five years earlier that I had other options like an IUD, that would have made it easier, I would have made a different choice. But there was no education. There was none of that."

The reason Allison had gone on birth control in the beginning was to manage her period. The IUD has eliminated the bad migraines and nausea she'd get every month, but she couldn't find much information or research on whether this form of birth control might help or hinder athletic performance or how it might impact her physiologically. That's a common issue for all athletes who are seeking birth control options. "When I was getting headaches and throwing up every month, it was very much a medical issue but because it dealt with my reproductive health, I had to jump through all these hoops to compete in my sport," she says. "And, well, I can't play if I'm pregnant, right?" Avoiding pregnancy, of course, is not the only reason for taking contraception; it can also help decrease bleeding, make the cycle shorter or more predictable, treat acne, or alleviate other period-related symptoms. But as more states pass legislation that restricts or bans abortion—including those that are home to most of the Southeastern Conference, as well as much of the Big 12 and Big Ten—education about birth control is vital.

Ironically, the Supreme Court overturned *Roe v. Wade* the day after we celebrated the fiftieth anniversary of when Title IX became law. Pro soccer star Megan Rapinoe tearfully spoke what so many people across the country felt that day. "It's oddly cruel for this to happen during this time of Title IX, celebrating this piece of legislation that gave so many women the opportunity to make our own choices about what we wanted to do with our lives," she said, adding, "and in the context of athletics, gave us the opportunity to pursue a unicorn talent to be professional athletes . . . or go to college and get an education." Rapinoe and five hundred other athletes, including Olympians, pros in the WNBA and NWSL, and hundreds of college athletes, had submitted an amicus brief in *Dobbs vs. Jackson Women's Health Organization*[2] (the Supreme Court decision that overturned *Roe*), including personal accounts about how reproductive freedom had been essential in gaining opportunities to participate in sports and to achieve their professional goals. Crissy Perham, a double-gold-medalist swimmer at the 1992 Olympics, detailed her unwanted pregnancy while on birth control during college. "I was on scholarship, I was just starting to succeed in my sport, and I didn't want to take a year off. I decided to have an abortion. I wasn't ready to be a mom, and having an abortion felt like I was given a second chance at life," she said.

An anonymous track and field athlete also described a situation that too many women find themselves in. By most estimates, one in five college women experience sexual assault each year.

> Many female teammates shared their experiences of sexual assault and rape with me during my time on the team. These experiences had extreme consequences on their mental health, athletic performances and seeped into all aspects of their everyday lives. For some of my teammates, the sexual violence they experienced was at the hands of our male teammates . . . these women had to face the recurring trauma of seeing their perpetrator every day at practice. If they were unable to access a safe and legal abortion after experiencing rape and were forced to carry a child to term the burden would have been unbearable.

Since the Supreme Court's decision in 2022, the NCAA and the leadership of most institutions have offered no guidance or training to coaches or staff about how to support an athlete who experiences an unplanned and unwanted pregnancy in states in which abortion is unavailable. One study, published in 2023 in the *Journal of Intercollegiate Sport*, found that of 146 female athletes at a large Division I university in the Midwest, 90 percent were unaware of the NCAA's policies on pregnancy, and 98 percent said they hadn't received any information from their athletic department.[3]

That tracks for coaches like Brooke, who says her athletic department has no protocol for staff members who might learn of an athlete's pregnancy. Another coach simply said, "I have no information on that." In fact, when we asked several NCAA coaches what policies they follow in the case of a pregnancy on the team, most had no guidelines to follow. "I would hope that my athletes would come to me in situations like this so we can talk about it and [they] can make a sound decision based on what they want to do," Brooke says.

While many people assume that women must experience deep regret, stress, and grief in choosing to abort an unwanted pregnancy, the research says otherwise. The Turnaway Study, an analysis of abortion from Advancing New Standards in Reproductive Health at the University of California San Francisco,[4] followed a thousand women across twenty-one states for five years to examine the similarities and differences between those who wanted and received an abortion versus those who wanted but were denied an abortion. Relief was the most commonly found emotion after receiving an abortion, and five years later, 97 percent said that the abortion was the right decision. "The bottom line is that abortion in and of itself does not cause mental health issues," says M. Antonia Biggs, PhD,[5] a psychologist and one of the leaders of the study.

The positive effects of bodily autonomy also extend to transgender and nonbinary people. A 2023 study followed three hundred transgender and nonbinary adolescents in the United States over two years and found that those who received gender-affirming hormones experienced less depression and anxiety and more satisfaction with life than before treatment.[6] This reinforces previous research that has found improved mental health outcomes for people who receive all kinds of gender-affirming care, a term that encompasses social, psychological, behavioral, and medical interventions that support a person's gender identity when it does not match the gender assigned at birth.

Layshia Clarendon, the WNBA's first openly transgender and nonbinary player, for example, publicly shared their joy in 2021 after getting top surgery, a procedure that removes breast tissue. "It's hard to put into words the feeling of seeing my chest for the first time free of breasts, seeing my chest the way I've always seen it, and feeling a sense of gender euphoria as opposed to gender dysphoria," they wrote on Instagram,[7] also adding, "I'm usually not scared to share news publicly but the amount of hate, myths & ignorance surrounding Trans and Non Binary people's existence actually had me debating sharing this joy . . . I want people to remember that my freedom is your freedom because none of us are free until we are all free!!!"

SUPPORTING ATHLETE CHOICES

Sara Vaughn, a professional marathon runner and two-time World Championships qualifier in the fifteen hundred meters, is on a mission to help pregnant and parenting NCAA athletes know their rights and feel more supported in accomplishing their dreams. She and her now husband, Brent Vaughn, faced challenges in 2006, when they were scholarship track and field athletes at the University of Colorado Boulder and Sara became unexpectedly pregnant with their daughter Kiki. Sara recalls that when they went to the campus health center to investigate what kind of care she could receive there, the nurse initially assumed they wanted to schedule an abortion. The dozen or so other female athletes who visited the center each semester had requested that option. But Sara, nineteen years old at the time, had decided to proceed with the pregnancy. It was uncharted territory for her and her coaches. She continued to compete during the indoor track season, but when she showed up to the team's study hall, she was turned away when the administrator didn't believe she belonged there as a visibly pregnant person.

Sara's coaches never discussed what would happen or how she could make a safe, healthy return to training and competition. Some professors demanded she return to class four days after giving birth, so she took her infant with her. She knew she needed to keep up her grades and return to practice as soon as possible to retain her scholarship, so she and Brent mapped out childcare duties between morning and night classes, study time, and running. Brent played poker to earn cash to keep them afloat. Grandparents traveled with them to help, and teammates held Kiki whenever they needed an extra set of hands. "I just assumed that I would try my best to come back as quickly as possible," Sara says. "I think part of my saving grace through the whole thing was my total naivety."

Sixteen years later, now with four children, the Vaughns know that athletes deserve a better way. They started the Vaughn Childcare Fund to help parenting student athletes complete their degrees by providing funds to pay for childcare, which is often the biggest obstacle that they face. The nonprofit organization is also providing education and mentoring to fill in the gaps on college campuses, where the NCAA estimates around 92 percent of universities lack written policy to guide responses to athlete pregnancies and parenting concerns. "The overwhelming emotion that I've heard from anybody who's experienced this is the pressure to either exit the university system if you're going to have a baby or get an abortion . . . they just feel like they don't have options," Sara says. "And that was pretty explicit with me, too. I had to really be like, 'No, actually, coach, I'm going to have this baby.'"

The NCAA offers a 107-page model policy[8] that was released in 2008 to help colleges form their own guidelines for caring for pregnant athletes. It states that athletes can't be excluded from their teams or denied scholarships because of "pregnancy, childbirth, false pregnancy, termination of pregnancy, or recovery therefrom." Under Title IX, students cannot be penalized for seeking, receiving, or recovering from a legal abortion. But in states where abortion is now illegal, the NCAA has not clarified its stance. It also remains unclear if helping an athlete travel to another state for an abortion is considered "aiding and abetting," which is also illegal in some regions.

The confusion leaves athletes in scary and overwhelming circumstances—unsure or unaware of their rights, like the option to take a medical redshirt (a year off from competition without losing a season of eligibility) so they can return to their scholarship position. "I hope they know that they're not alone in whatever decision they make," Sara says. "It all comes back to awareness and letting people know their options and rights."

FIGHTING FOR THEIR DREAMS

Athletes who plan to start their families during their careers also face real challenges. The decision often comes down to timing pregnancy against the competitive schedule. Sometimes it entails delaying pregnancy until the end of a career with methods like egg freezing, though such options are expensive, often not fully covered by insurance, and not guaranteed to work, of course. Some decide to adopt, while others face fertility challenges. Others consider the implications of breastfeeding on athletic performance and the reality of work-related travel. The dream is creating a world where women can plan pregnancy if and when it works best for them—without derailing their athletic careers. Starting a family is never a simple process, and it's full of difficult decisions that male counterparts rarely need to consider. This is why many female athletes are devoting a lot of time and energy to demanding parental protections, making headway on behalf of all athletes who wish to start their families during the peak of their careers.

Alex Morgan, a decorated pro soccer star who gave birth to her daughter in 2020, has been an outspoken advocate for such athletes. Through collective bargaining with the players' union, the NWSL now offers eight weeks of parental leave, and Morgan has also pointed out other ways in which clubs and teams can help athletes remain successful on the field while parenting, like providing accommodations, meals, and travel expenses for caregivers (like nannies and babysitters). "You shouldn't own a team if you can't (financially) support your players,"[9] Alex once tweeted in response to a question about the limited resources that organizations may have for new parents.

Alex's US teammate Becky Sauerbrunn shared in 2022 that she had decided to freeze her eggs at age thirty-six. In that process, she had to take a leave from training—she told the On Her Turf podcast[10] that "broaching the subject with the national team, that was kind of terrifying. I was basically cramming this month-long process in between two national team camps." Nonetheless, the reality that Becky was facing about her fertility and career timeline wasn't foreign to any athlete. She had been inspired to talk about it after learning about the WNBA's agreement with its players association in 2019, which included the option for a $20,000 reimbursement each year for costs related to adoption, surrogacy, egg freezing, or fertility/infertility treatment. "I didn't want that added pressure when trying to decide the future of my career," Becky told *On Her Turf*. "As someone who is an older athlete . . . I often have to think, 'Will I want to start a family?'"

The lack of widespread maternal support is a reflection of the lack of safety net for all parents in the United States, of course. In 2018, sprinter Allyson Felix, the most decorated track and field athlete of all time (thirty-two medals between the Olympics and World Championships before her 2021 retirement), trained in the dark, predawn hours to hide her pregnancy from her then sponsor, Nike, with whom she was in the midst of renegotiating her contract. The brand was already proposing to reduce her payment by 70 percent and was refusing pregnancy protection, she said in a *New York Times* op-doc.[11] At the time, Nike and other brands traditionally cut payment to athletes who were unable to compete for any reason—pregnancy and postpartum recovery included.

Allyson delivered her daughter at thirty-two weeks by emergency cesarean section, after suffering life-threatening preeclampsia. As her daughter spent her first months in the NICU, Allyson continued to hide her news. During that time, she also began to learn more about Black maternal-health-care disparities, reading the research that plainly shows that health care providers spend less time with Black mothers and dismiss their symptoms more often—one of the main reasons they are three times more likely to die from pregnancy-related causes than white women. Just a year earlier, Serena Williams had her own harrowing experience while giving birth by c-section. Prone to blood clots, Serena told doctors that she was concerned she was having a pulmonary embolism. The healthcare team initially denied her request for a CT scan and a blood thinner, assuming she was in pain or just confused. Finally, after an ultrasound of her legs didn't reveal anything, they ordered the CT scan that displayed clots on her lungs.

Allyson has since testified on Capitol Hill on behalf of Black mothers, detailing the racial bias in their health care. And just as Nike released a "Dream Maternity" campaign, showcasing athletes as mothers, she and fellow pro runners Kara Goucher and Alysia Montaño went public in the *New York Times*[12] about how the brand and other corporations exploited their motherhood without pay or protections. Weeks later, Nike was among the brands that announced new policies for sponsored athletes who became pregnant while under contract, guaranteeing payment and bonuses for eighteen months. Allyson ultimately signed a new contract with Athleta, the women's apparel brand, as the company's first sponsored athlete. It led the company to a partnership with Simone Biles, too.

During a press conference after her final Olympics in Tokyo, Allyson reflected on her decision to take a stand not just for herself but for every mother, no matter what her career path. "I feel like it's definitely been a journey for me to get to the point where I guess I have the courage to do so and I think that just comes with experiences in life," she said. "I'm happy I was able to get to this place because there's so much that needs to be done and I think it was just my own experience of going through it that really opened my eyes to all of it."

Women face exceptional expectations as mothers—from society and from within themselves, too. The guilt of leaving their children with other caregivers to pursue their careers, unable to be in two places at the same time, is real. Just like moms in all professions, they want to do what they love and take care of their children, too. Athletes deal with the same challenges that all new parents face, including childcare access and costs, breastfeeding logistics as they return to work, and other factors like postpartum depression, for example, that can sideline their return to competition.

And it's not surprising that so many athletes want to return to training quickly—becoming a parent takes them out of the structure, routines, and some validation that they've always thrived on. While exercise has been shown to give some protection against postpartum depression, athletes are not immune from experiencing symptoms. Serena Williams explained in 2018 that she was going through "tough personal stuff" as she returned to the US Open just three months after giving birth. Mostly, she said on Instagram, she didn't feel like she was a good mom, but talking about it with her mother, sister, and friends allowed her to realize that what she was going through was normal. "I work a lot, I train, and I'm trying to be the best athlete I can be. However, that means although I have been with her every day of her life, I'm not around as much as I would like to be. Most of you moms deal with the same thing," Serena wrote. "I'm here to say: If you are having a rough day or week—it's OK—I am, too!!!"[13]

Alysia, an Olympian and three-time World Championships bronze medalist in the eight hundred meters, and mother of three, has long advocated for pregnant athletes, gaining notoriety in 2014 when she competed at the national track and field championships while eight months pregnant, in an effort to show women that they could become mothers and still have successful athletic careers. She went on to win two national championships in the months after giving birth to her first child and represented the United States in Beijing at the world championships, where she pumped breast milk and shipped it home for her daughter. Alysia started writing legislation that protected pregnant athletes' access to health insurance from the US Olympic Committee—at the time, insurance was stripped from women who had to take a break from competing.

On Mother's Day 2020, Alysia launched a nonprofit organization called &Mother to help drive change in "a working world that has historically discriminated against, dismissed, and undervalued motherhood, starting with professional athletics."[14] Among the initiatives the organization has undertaken: a grant program to help athletes cover family expenses or mental health support, sponsorships up to $10,000 for new moms chasing goals like the Olympic Trials, and partnering with corporations to help breastfeeding Olympians store or ship their breast milk from the 2021 Tokyo Games. &Mother has also set up lactation stations at major athletic events and provided free childcare for competing athletes.

It's organizations like Alysia's and the Vaughns' that are filling in the major gaps that the systems have long neglected, making it possible for women to worry less and compete more. It's also the courage of the athletes who are openly sharing their stories that are compelling leagues and sport governing federations, as well as corporate sponsors, to pay attention, allowing more athletes a bit more space to consider parenthood and know that they will have the support to return to training and competition.

From Serena dealing with postpartum changes to the middle school softball player figuring out her cycle, the choices that female athletes make each and every day about their reproductive health are complicated, politicized, often fraught with fear, shame, and guilt, and made in unnecessary isolation and suffering. If we're serious about supporting and improving the mental health of girls and women in sports, we have to start by removing the restrictions and stigmas that society has placed on their bodies and personal health care decisions.

Chapter Thirteen

HEALING IN THE AFTERMATH OF SPORTS

Participating in athletics has a lifelong impact and many
athletes eventually need to process trauma.

Emily, the swimmer at the SEC D-I program who we first introduced in chapter 3, has developed a coping strategy when her thoughts turn to the days when she and her teammates sat by the pool while their coach berated them for disappointing performances. "You need to work harder! You're not trying hard enough! This is how I feed my family!" he'd scream. Now Emily envisions herself on the deck encased in a plastic bubble. Her coach's words hit the protective orb and bounce right off. She tells herself, "His anger is not for me."

Since she left the program, Emily has sought help to figure out why it sometimes still haunts her. She still remembers that daily feeling of panic if she didn't arrive at the pool forty-five minutes early. She recalls the day her coaches ruthlessly cut women from the team midpractice, pulling them from a set and sending them to the locker room in tears, only hours before the NCAA transfer deadline. She remembers how the older swimmers forced excessive drinking on the younger ones at parties, the hazing and intimidation, and harassment from members of the men's team that she, more than once, had feared would turn into assault. And when she feels the anxiety and emotions rushing back, she taps her fingers together and reminds herself to be calm. With the help of her therapist, she's learned that closing her eyes and finding that peace makes those memories feel smaller. Her breathing deepens and her heart rate decreases. Emily can mentally go to a better, safer place. "There's a meadow and creek beside me. It's a magical spot where my brain slows down," she says. "I don't feel like I'm spiraling."

Emily has family and friends who support her alongside her mental-health care provider, as she heals from the anxiety still vivid from that chapter of her collegiate career. She also leans on her faith. She still remembers sobbing in the kitchen of her parents' home, explaining how much stress swimming—her ticket to a college education—was causing her. At that point, her mother encouraged her to seek help from a mental-health care provider. Emily was fortunate to begin therapy while still navigating the unhealthy dynamic of her program. She was able to recognize that her experience and the ensuing emotions were real and valid—something so many athletes never realize, or at least not until after they've left their athletic careers behind. "Coaches' language has so much power," Emily says. "And you start to bargain with yourself because that coach has something that every athlete wants: success. You listen to what they say so you can be successful. My coach was a certified counselor—he had his psychology degree displayed in his office. In my mind, I could trust him. Now I just think that he understood what he was doing to people. But back then I felt like I was crazy."

Over time, she's learned about "big-T" and "little-t trauma." Like so many of us, when Emily thought about trauma, she associated it with a massive, terrible event like assault, gun violence, or a life-threatening car crash. She didn't understand that she had experienced a different form of trauma, a form that she carried with her from spending years in a toxic sports environment. As we touched on in earlier chapters, trauma can result from a single event, like an assault or an accident, for example, or it can come from a long-term, chronic pattern like neglect, bullying, racism, or physical or emotional abuse. According to the National Center for Post-Traumatic Stress Disorder (PTSD), more than half of all women will be exposed to at least one traumatic event in their lifetime,[1] and research published in the *European Journal of Psychotraumatology* reveals that women experience PTSD (a diagnosed anxiety disorder in reaction to physical injury or severe mental or emotional distress) at two to three times the rate that men do.[2]

Many female athletes emerge from sports without a fully developed perspective on what they experienced through the years of training, competing, and devoting so much of their lives to the pursuit. For some people, it's only with the benefit of hindsight that they can identify forms of mistreatment, misogyny, racism, homophobia, or transphobia they endured. Others don't realize they've developed an unhealthy relationship with food or distorted body image, for example, until they are no longer part of teams that normalize or demand it of them. Even concussions and other devastating injuries can lead to traumatic responses that take time to recognize and process. Healing may take years and can involve resentment, confusion, shame, embarrassment, and anger. It might involve rewiring the defenses that were created to cope with the harm. But it doesn't matter where or when the healing process starts; it's just important to begin.

We know it's not that easy, though. We live in a society that regularly does not believe or even respond to women when they describe what has happened to them. And women are well aware of what happens when they speak up and a perpetrator or institution is held accountable. Offenders deny the behavior, attack the individual who is confronting that behavior, and reverse the role of victim and offender (the offender assumes the role of "falsely accused" and attacks the accuser's credibility). Experts call it DARVO ("deny, attack, and reverse victim and offender"). No wonder so many women choose to remain quiet: one study found that 44 percent of perpetrators deny their offenses and call their accuser "crazy," and a study on violence in sports from the University of Delaware's Center for the Study and Prevention of

Gender-Based Violence found that in 75 percent of cases, the accused athlete or coach was allowed to continue to work or compete, regardless of whether they were charged, arrested, or convicted.[3]

We also know that sports culture encourages athletes to suppress pain and emotions while it celebrates the obedient (or "coachable"), making it challenging for athletes to acknowledge painful memories or question the people and systems in which they had placed their trust. Jennifer Freyd, PhD, a scholar best known for her theories on betrayal trauma, described it as "when people or institutions on which a person depends for survival significantly violate that person's trust or well-being."[4] An athlete relies on coaches, athletic departments, universities, and the sport itself for a sense of belonging and community, a place to develop skills, a chance to get an education, and, of course, a means of learning how to thrive and win under pressure. A coach, school, or program hold enormous power in the relationship, and many athletes resort to "betrayal blindness" while they continue participating to preserve the relationships, institutions, and social systems that they depend on. In abusive situations like those we discussed in chapter 6, for example, athletes may choose to stay in the situations to continue to receive scholarship money or because the mistreatment has been normalized to the degree that they don't realize until later that it is inappropriate and harmful.

Libby, for example, traveled the world as an elite cyclist, and her career looked like a dream from the outside. Getting to see the far reaches of the globe while pursuing the sport she loved was an enviable position. But what nobody saw—what never made the Instagram grid or highlight reel—was how her coach chastised her female teammates and her. Libby was called lazy and slow. The coach, a man who led the European-based group, would get in her face and scream how embarrassed he was by her performance. He'd dissect the women's bodies and label them "soft" when they didn't meet his expectations.

For years, Libby chalked up the coach's behavior to cultural differences. That's how she got through it. She'd justify the abuse as language just lost in translation. The more he screamed, the harder Libby trained.

She craved the pain of the workouts to numb herself to the agony of the abuse. When she left the sport, she assumed she had left the entire ordeal behind her, but it took several years postretirement for Libby to identify what she had experienced and was still experiencing: trauma. Exercise triggered flashbacks, especially cycling. So she sold all of her bikes, which once represented joy and purpose but now evoked anxiety and panic. Libby also became distrustful of others and isolated. Her therapist suggested a link between how she was feeling and her experience in sports. Libby hadn't thought of that connection; she had sought help based on her feelings and emotions.

We've seen this scenario play out in our own offices—former athletes who have disconnected from their feelings until we touch on a trigger spot. Again, the athlete mindset requires a level of separation from emotion that doesn't work well when you're trying to improve mental health. Dissociating is required in sports, but it's problematic in life. The goal, however, is to learn how to feel the whole spectrum of emotions, from joy to heartache. Healing feels tricky because duality is challenging. You may feel gratitude for having had the opportunity to compete at the highest levels, but you may resent the harm and confusion that came with it. Both emotions are true, and you can experience them at the exact same time.

Libby underwent a psychotherapy treatment called Eye Movement Desensitization and Reprocessing (EMDR), which alleviates distress associated with traumatic memories by helping you access the negative events and reprocess what you remember. A therapist will ask you to remember a traumatic scene and focus on the feelings and sensations that come up while quickly moving your eyes left to right, mimicking REM sleep (this movement helps evoke emotions related to the trauma). Over time, the emotions connected to the memories decrease in intensity and you're able to replace negative thoughts with more positive associations. Before treatment like EMDR, however, you have to work on developing effective coping skills and trust in yourself. A clinician will assess that readiness before beginning EMDR (we encourage discussions with providers who can help you determine the best route forward for you).

After seven months of this treatment, Libby finally felt at peace; her memories of her pro sports career didn't cause fear, panic, or anxiety anymore, and she was even able to enjoy cycling again. Ultimately, the work helped her untangle the pressure to win races from the pleasure of pedaling to see the world around her. She did this by homing in on her body signals and the early signs that indicated a trauma response. She had GI issues while competing, and she learned to listen to her body's feedback. Rather than ignoring triggers and the discomfort of cycling memories, she can talk about them and think about that period of her life without spiraling.

COMMON TRAUMA RESPONSES

Regardless of what type of trauma an athlete has gone through, it's common to experience reactions afterward like stress, fear, or anger. Sometimes a person who has been through trauma can't stop thinking about it. For athletes, often the trauma was a daily event, sustained through a significant portion of their lives. Other times, trauma can cause physical and emotional responses to triggers that might seem unexpected—but after you identify what those triggers are, you're better able to cope with them. Here are a few common reactions to trauma, according to the National Center for PTSD[5]:

- Loss of hope for the future
- Feeling distant or having lack of concern for others
- Startling easily at sudden noises
- Feeling on guard and alert all the time
- Experiencing dreams and memories that are upsetting
- Having problems at work or school
- Avoiding people and places related to your traumatic experience

Physical reactions to trauma:

- Stomach upset and trouble eating
- Problems sleeping while also feeling tired
- Increased heart rate, rapid breathing, feeling shaky
- Sweating
- Headaches, sometimes brought on by thinking about the trauma
- Ceasing exercise, healthy diet, safe sex, or regular health care
- Using alcohol or other substances or eating too much or too little
- Letting ongoing medical problems worsen

Emotional reactions to trauma:

- Feeling nervous, helpless, fearful, and sad
- Feeling shocked, numb, or unable to feel love or joy
- Irritability and angry outbursts
- Blaming yourself or having negative views of yourself
- Inability to trust others, getting into fights, or trying to control everything
- Withdrawing, or feeling rejected or abandoned
- Feeling detached and not wanting intimacy

WHERE TO BEGIN

Amy, the runner at the small Christian university in the south who we first met in chapter 5, realized soon after she graduated that she could no longer live in the college town, which is also where she grew up and where her family still resides. She had come forward to the university leadership about her emotional abuse, filed Title IX reports, and had taken the matter to the US Center for SafeSport, detailing what she and other teammates had experienced during their tenure on the cross-country and track and field teams, which included food- and body-shaming, harassment, bullying, and neglect. She had been sexually assaulted during her first year of college and subsequently suffered anxiety, depression, and a suicide attempt—and as a result, she had difficulty meeting her coach's performance expectations. When she explained why she was struggling, he did not offer empathy or help; he told her that subsequent injuries and health problems were all in her head and that she was letting the team down, she says. After graduation, she made her story public, and dozens of other former and current athletes and university staff corroborated it, even adding similar stories of their own related to bullying, injuries, and eating disorders exacerbated by body composition testing and the coach's food shaming. Still, Amy coped with backlash by those who sided with the coach and the university, an institution she says plays a prominent role in the community.

For Amy, getting a fresh start in a new city was a key step in the process of healing from the disordered eating that had continued for a time after college. "I just wanted to be as small as possible. I couldn't handle being seen or being noticed and I just really wanted to make myself disappear, in a way," Amy says. "Moving away was really necessary for me. I couldn't go to the grocery store without feeling concerned that I'd run into somebody." She moved out of state and started noticing how much relief came just by relocating, along with talk therapy and a low dose of antidepressant medication. During her time in college, her coaches had impressed upon her that nobody on the team wanted to be friends with her because she was depressed, which eventually led her to believe that she'd never have many friends. Moving away showed her that wasn't true. "They'd keep telling me that nobody wanted to be around me and that I brought everybody down and it just stuck with me," Amy says. "Forming new friendships in a new city has been really hard for me but has let me see that people do enjoy being around me and I can have healthy relationships."

Although running had once played a big part in Amy's life, she's still reluctant to train again. While she was competing in college, acceptance from her coaches and many teammates hinged on her performances, and over time she was conditioned to ignore her instincts about everything from hunger signals to injuries. She still hasn't fully regained confidence in herself to make healthy decisions, so she has taken a step back from running for now. "I was taught to not trust myself while at the same time I was putting all my trust in this school, these coaches, and the people around me and I felt pretty betrayed," Amy says.

Lauren, who ran for the same university and coach as Amy but ten years earlier, wasn't able to break those cycles. Today, Lauren is back in treatment for a relapse of her eating disorder, spurred by a fracture in her foot that has prevented her from exercising while it healed. Now in her forties, she still traces a lot of her current problematic habits to her time on the cross-country team. In one of her group therapy sessions in May 2023, she talked about some of the practices that were ingrained by her coach. She still skips dessert and any drinks with calories—two things that were not allowed while she was competing. "I hear his voice numerous times to this day," she says. "He says, 'You're lazy, you're lazy, you're lazy.'"

The female athletes we spoke with told us that at the time, they thought what they were experiencing during their sports careers was standard—the unspoken price they agreed to pay to compete. Emotional abuse was normalized. Coping with big injuries in isolation or training through them was part of the deal. Body-shaming, weigh-ins, and fat testing were strategies to help athletes perform better. Nobody else seemed bothered by any of it, so all of it must have been appropriate, right? So why, these athletes ask, do we feel the magnitude of it now? The short answer is that we all process our experiences in our own time. Some athletes are quick to recognize what happened, and others take longer to acknowledge it (or sometimes never do). The right time is whenever the athlete chooses and feels ready. From a mental health perspective, we know that readiness makes all the difference. You can't force someone to turn toward healing. And a person's readiness can shift over time. It's important to honor the timeline of every person turning toward their own trauma and recognize that healing looks different for everyone.

To be sure, many people come away from sports carrying a heavy load of emotions, confusion, and shame with them—if that's your experience, you are far from alone. We all see the headlines and read the breaking news about a fired coach or a program under investigation, but we rarely follow up with the people whose lives are forever changed because of how they were treated in sports. The good news? The human spirit is remarkable and resilient. We are wired for survival, and we forge on despite (or even because of) whatever happens. But those who are coping with trauma must realize that they can't simply forget about their experiences. Healing involves remembering. When we go through trauma, the brain changes. The part of the brain that regulates thinking and emotions becomes underactive while the part that detects fear is overactive—to return the mind to a healthy condition, we have to work hard to change it again. But we know healing is possible because we see it all the time in our work.

Physiologically, the body also experiences trauma long after the initial events took place. Most of us have heard about the "fight or flight" response, which is an automatic reaction to a situation that is stressful or frightening. It's our body's way of helping us survive. Our sympathetic nervous system activates a chain reaction that increases our heart rate, increases our respiration, and blood circulation is directed to our brains and muscles. Adrenaline and cortisol, the primary stress hormones, surge (this is a good thing when we need it; it's what helps us survive dangerous situations). Then, when the stress subsides, our parasympathetic nervous system helps return our body functions to normal. The problem is that when the body is exposed to long-term trauma, it keeps producing cortisol, which increases the risk of conditions like anxiety, depression, heart disease, insomnia, and loss of the ability to focus. In addition to fight and flight, people also have two other responses to trauma triggers, which we discussed in chapter 6: freeze and fawn. The freeze response is exactly what it sounds like—a person just stops reacting and hopes she won't be noticed. A fawn response is typical in cases of abuse, when an athlete becomes overly compliant and seeks to please the abuser to avoid conflict.

In our therapy work, we sometimes start treatment by asking the athlete to write letters or journal entries that allow the athlete to describe what she's feeling and the questions she has, which illuminate more information about her fears. Often, the information we're searching for seems more daunting when it's internalized; getting it down on paper allows the athlete to externalize and explore what she's feeling. It can feel intense as the nervous system becomes overloaded by feelings that involve fear and betrayal. For so long, an athlete has relied on coping strategies to get away from those emotions, sometimes by using substances, dissociation (disconnecting from thoughts or memories), or just by looking for distractions. Looking inward and surfacing emotions that are connected in the past are how we learn more about them, in the present.

Though we understand that therapy is not accessible to everybody and it also seems like a daunting proposition to undertake, it is especially helpful in trauma recovery. It's a place where you're believed and supported as you heal. An effective therapist will help you discover your path forward, help you overcome the obstacles along the way, and provide a safe environment as you begin to understand how your nervous system reacts to talking about traumatic events. Therapy, no doubt, requires a lot of difficult work. You have to commit to accountability, reflection, and growth. It's a challenging process. One client who was beginning to discuss her trauma said it made her want to run away, adding, "My body is on the verge of a panic attack." In this case, we worked on self-soothing strategies—for athletes who have been conditioned to ignore their body's cues, it can be especially challenging sometimes to tune into these signals and connect with themselves. But over time, they can learn to self-regulate, managing the stress on their own.

Matching with the right therapist is important—somebody who understands the role of trauma and some understanding of athletics is valuable. A friend's well-intentioned referral may not be the best fit; you're the only one who can determine if your relationship with your therapist feels right. And if it doesn't, don't give up. Even as therapists, we know that not all of us are the right fit for everyone. You deserve healing, and finding the person who can go on that journey with you may take time. Keep going.

Shaylah, a high-performing pole-vaulter who competed for a large program in the Southwest, still sometimes believes that her body isn't good enough, years after retiring from a semipro career. It stems from an injury early in her NCAA career, competing through a stress fracture that landed her in a boot and crutches for an entire summer. She couldn't cross-train or maintain any physical activity for months, and she arrived for fall training ten pounds heavier. Her coach was furious. He began putting her through weekly weigh-ins, and her body composition became the center of their conversations for several years. In post-collegiate competition, her coach asked her to keep a food log, which she refused to do because it provoked anxiety. Yet another coach encouraged her to eat her meals on a children's plate to reduce her portions. As she picked up a few modeling gigs, Shaylah was told she'd be more marketable if she "leaned out."

It took Shaylah several years and some therapy before she started developing strategies to overcome her guilt associated with food and eating. "The inside voice is so mean," she says. "I had to stop ignoring the inside voice and interact with it, trace it back, and remind myself that I am not 'Shaylah the pole-vaulter' anymore and that is OK. I need to learn who I am now and who I want to be in the future and correct the voice that constantly compares me to who I was as an athlete."

COPING WITH TRAUMA

One of the most effective ways of treating trauma is with a mental-health care provider who is qualified to help you develop strategies that will change your thinking patterns. If your distress is disrupting relationships, work, or daily life, it's best to seek help from a therapist, mostly so you don't have to go about coping and healing on your own.

Therapy is tightly bound to individual cultures. Athletes who are more accustomed to community and collectivism, for example, might be drawn to other ways of healing. Historically, people have found many other ways to achieve the same goals, through practices rooted in Indigenous beliefs and traditions or shamanism, for example. Not everybody requires treatment for trauma—some people can recover on their own, in time. Here are a few strategies that we recommend, along with the American Psychological Association,[6] when you're coping with traumatic stress:

Seek support. Identify the people in your life who you can trust to talk about your experiences, your feelings, and will support you by validating what happened and how it has caused you distress.

Trust yourself. If something feels unsettling or you notice a change in feelings, thoughts, or behaviors, trust it. You do not have to wait for concrete data to justify why you are feeling the way you are.

Honor your feelings. Athletes are pros at pushing pain aside, but to overcome traumatic stress you have to think about what happened and find healthy ways to cope with it. Avoidance, whether it's by sleeping excessively, isolating yourself, or using substances, won't get you back to a healthy state. Talk to your loved ones and write down your emotions. And if it feels like you need help to get started, try finding a therapist.

Be curious. When you have responses to events, thoughts, or circumstances, allow yourself to notice what you are feeling and question why.

Take care of yourself. Engage in activities that you find peaceful, like art, music, meditation, walking, or just spending time moving in nature. Eat nourishing food and try to get quality sleep every night if possible.

Create a plan. Determine what healing means to you and the best mode of accessing that support. Share your feelings with your support network, a mental health provider, and/or your doctors. Increase the time spent engaging in activities and rituals that further connect you to yourself, like nature, art, or music, for example.

> **Take your time.** Symptoms of distress may take time to improve and often progress isn't linear. You may feel like you have already done your healing work and the next thing you know, symptoms pop up again. That is normal. During different times in our lives, including developmental and life cycle stages, we have different needs.

LONG-TERM CONSEQUENCES

It may have taken place thirty years ago, but for one NCAA Division I swimmer who started at a major Southeast program before transferring to a Southwest university, the effects are still vivid. Blair* remembers the culture of substance-use disorder, sexual and emotional abuse, and "the whole gamut" of circumstances she and her teammates endured throughout her collegiate career. "If you wanted to be on the 'A' relay, you had to sleep with the coach," she says. "Some of us quit. Some of us stuck it out. Some of us transferred."

Among the common practices on the team were "pizza and purge parties." On Friday nights, the women would get together, order a lot of pizza, eat as much as they could, and then throw it up. They did the same when the team stopped at Olive Garden while traveling to and from meets. They were hungry from the intense training but feared joining what the coach called the "fat club," which entailed running the stadium steps after practice when an athlete didn't meet the target number on the scale. "We wanted to eat, but we knew we needed to be ready for Saturday morning practice and weigh-in," Blair recalls.

For thirty years after graduation, Blair couldn't go near a pool. Even the smell of chlorine would trigger traumatic memories—only after she had children did she get back in the water, finally able to separate the sport from the abusive coaches and administrators who perpetuated a harmful and toxic culture. "I didn't just get over it," Blair says. Despite trying different therapists and treatments like hypnosis, she still purges sometimes or tries intermittent fasting. "I still have a lot of issues with food," she admits. During her time competing at the collegiate level, the purging and weight-loss behaviors weren't secretive. The administrators and coaching staff knew what the athletes were doing and didn't condemn it, so it was normalized and often even glamorized. It ingrained the behavior and conditioning in athletes like Blair, who has gone to great lengths to overcome it.

Many former athletes find themselves experiencing shame in asking for help because decades have passed since they retired from their sports. It seems strange or even embarrassing to admit that they still grapple with the conditions and unhealthy habits they developed back then; they feel like they should have been able to "move on" by now. Whether the harm was caused last week or thirty years ago, the pain doesn't have an end point. Trauma doesn't go away—the key is to learn to live with it in a different way than you did before. Healing may seem mythical, but it is possible. As you learn the cues and your responses to them, you can change the feedback loop. As Nicole Spreadborough, LPC at Thrive Mental Health, shares, "You came up with strategies that helped the intolerable become tolerable in the moment and those are defense mechanisms that have protected the parts of us that hold the trauma."

Blair has relied mostly on self-healing, she says, trying to stay away from drug and alcohol use. What has made the most difference for her is discovering that she's not alone. "What has helped the most is reading personal stories from those who went through similar traumas and wrote about it," Blair says. "I sometimes think I'll write about it, but then change my mind because it's too dark and just spurs negative energy all around."

After she went public with her own story, Amy felt that same sort of kinship with others. She heard from dozens of former runners in her college program who had gone through the same kind of experiences with the same coach, ten or more years earlier. She also heard from prominent athletes across the country who offered empathy and support. Though the camaraderie helps validate what happened, Amy also finds it sad and infuriating that nothing has been done to protect athletes from further harm. She feels that most systems would rather protect the legacy of successful coaches than tend to the long-term impact that their behavior has had on their athletes. "I mean, there are so many examples of it—people who have been in different programs, have experienced abuse themselves, and some of them have seen change in their program but most of them haven't. We're able to really connect with that," she says. "I used to think, 'Who do I have to be for anyone to care? What do I have to have accomplished for anyone to make change happen? How bad would it have had to be?'"

Though the journey through trauma is individual, it is often the systems—and the institutions that protect them—that keep us stuck. The women we spoke to were universally worried about coming off as weak or whiny, but the way to take your power back is by doing the work to heal. It takes tremendous strength to confront trauma, but it is possible and can lead to renewed safety, relief, and empowerment.

Chapter Fourteen

AFTER SPORTS: WHAT COMES NEXT?

Planned or unplanned, voluntary or involuntary, departure
from sports comes with mixed emotions and sometimes grief.

Many athletes began their love affair with athletics so early in life
they barely remember a time without weekend tournaments,
after-school practices, and social outings with their teammates. But no
matter how old we were when we kicked our first soccer ball, made our
first basket, or ran our first race, sports have become a special part of us.
They're what we do and, for a time, they're also a big part of who we
are. During our most formative years, sports offered friendship, routines, validation, community, achievement, belonging, and more. It's
only natural that when our time as athletes comes to an end, we can
feel all kinds of emotions, ranging from relief to grief.

Common endpoints for athletes include high school or college
graduation—and for the elite set, usually sometime in their twenties or
thirties. No matter what the end date is, we know that athletes across
all ability levels and age groups struggle when the structure and depend-
ability of sports participation is gone.

The transition can be even harder for those who don't get the fairy-
tale ending they wanted—instead of winning the state title or an

Olympic gold medal or something in between, they lost that final match, or were cut from the team, or sustained major injuries. Meggie, who is now a mother and a 911 dispatcher in Colorado, vividly remembers her bumpy exit from collegiate competition. She had started playing soccer when she was five years old, and it didn't take long for coaches to identify her talent. As a youth player, she shot through the ranks of club teams and travel leagues and even a semipro group, with a singular focus on getting a scholarship to a Division I school—and the offer from a Big Ten program fulfilled that dream. Unfortunately, the reality of playing in the NCAA didn't match her vision. Meggie tore her medial collateral ligament (MCL) in the preseason during her first year, one of nine players who were injured likely due to the intense nature of the training. She was supposed to recover for twelve weeks, but the coach pulled her off her medical redshirt for the final two games, burning a year of her eligibility.

Nevertheless, Meggie was confident in her return to play as a defender the following year. She was in the best fitness of her life, she thought, and was making big contributions to the team. However, over the summer, she and others who were on the starting lineup were replaced with the first-year players that the new coach had recruited. Meggie wondered what she was doing so far away from home if she wasn't going to play anymore. So she moved back closer to her family and transferred to a fledgling DI program. "It felt like going back to rec soccer, so I ultimately ended up quitting," Meggie says. "The first six months of my transition out of sport felt great. Nobody is yelling at me. I can do whatever I want, whenever I want. But then I was completely lost. I only went to school to play soccer. I didn't know what career path I was going to take. I had no path at all."

With the loss of NCAA soccer, Meggie lost herself, too. She finished school and earned a degree in sociology, but in her personal life, she clung to an unhealthy relationship for five years. She struggled to figure out how to replace the addictive adrenaline rush that soccer always afforded her. She tried community coed leagues, which helped a little bit, but not enough. "You still think of yourself as an athlete, but you have a sense of embarrassment that you aren't who you were back then," she says. It was an email from her father, a firefighter, letting her know about a job opening as a 911 dispatcher that helped put Meggie in a position to move on. From the beginning, she wanted to become the best dispatcher ever—the one that all the firefighters wanted on the radio. Essentially, she was bringing the same drive to "win" on the field into the workplace and soon advanced to supervisory positions. Meggie also met her husband, a police officer, and now they are raising three children. "When I had my daughter in 2016, my whole world flipped upside down; this little being depends on me and that is a whole new loyalty and love," Meggie says. "Parenting softened me a lot. All my life I was the most aggressive soccer player. I was dirty and I played hard. That was who I was. I liked to be tough and gritty and I never cried."

Looking back, Meggie wishes she had been given the opportunity to meet with a mental-health care provider when she was leaving soccer so she had a better idea what to expect and the challenges she might encounter. "It would have been such a gift to learn these coping skills or at least be given some information on the things you might feel and go through," she says. "I just traded one thing for the other."

What Meggie went through is not unique. In our many conversations with women across all sports, most were surprised by the heavy emotions they felt after moving on. With such laser focus on big goals, lots of athletes never planned for what would come next. Another common postsports challenge? So many women say they have struggled with their body image as their physique and fitness levels changed. They didn't know how to exercise merely as a healthy habit; without the pursuit of competition, practice times, and training schedules, they didn't know where to start. The lack of steady endorphins sometimes also resulted in new levels of mood swings.

It's not as easy as just hanging up the cleats and calling it for good for most athletes—not even for Serena Williams, who announced her retirement in an essay she wrote for *Vogue* in 2022. She felt that to have another child, she would have to end her tennis career at age forty, yet, she admitted having conflicting feelings about the decision. "I'm going to be honest. There is no happiness in this topic for me," she wrote. "I know it's not the usual thing to say, but I feel a great deal of pain. It's the hardest thing I could ever imagine. I hate it. I hate that I have to be at this crossroads. I keep saying to myself, I wish it could be easy for me, but it's not. I'm torn: I don't want it to be over, but at the same time I'm ready for what's next."

On August 22, 2023, Serena announced the birth of her second child, Adira River Ohanian.[1]

NAVIGATING THE TRANSITION TO POST-SPORT LIFE

Some athletes walk away from the final game feeling a sense of excitement for what's next. Or relief that it's over. But more often, players can feel a sense of loss, grief, and confusion. Remember that it takes time to move from one phase of life to another—give yourself grace and try some of these strategies to help your transition:

- Give yourself permission to grieve or struggle with the change. A transition brings up all kinds of feelings and new routines. It's OK to take some time as you make these changes.
- Maintain a schedule that includes quality sleep, nourishing meals, and physical activity, to help keep mood swings in check, alleviate stress, and give a sense of routine.
- Try a daily practice of listening to your body, a meditation practice when you tune into your body and notice areas of pain, tension, or anything unusual, which helps you feel more connected to your physical and emotional self.
- Talk to former teammates who are going through or have gone through retirement. Sharing the ups and downs will remind you

that you're not alone. Chances are, whatever you're feeling, others are, too.

- Consider coaching a youth program to offer your expertise and stay connected to the sport.
- Join a local club and pursue a different activity like running, cycling, rock climbing, or tennis, for example. Expand your social network by trying something you've never done before.
- If you're feeling persistent sadness or symptoms of depression, find support from a mental-health care professional.

CLAIMING IDENTITY

Serena went on to write that the only person she was able to discuss the end of her career with was her therapist; in fact, she decided against using the word "retirement" altogether, opting instead for "evolving," or "discovering a different, but just as exciting Serena." It was an off-limits conversation with basically anybody else, including her husband, because it brought on such immense sadness.

You don't have to carry the moniker "Greatest of All Time" in your sport to feel similar sorrow when it's over. Among the general population, research on the prevalence of depression among new retirees is lacking, but a 2020 meta-analysis of eleven studies found that one in three people report mental health symptoms upon retiring from their careers.[2] While athletes' retirements are much different (coming at a younger age, for one, and likely involve moving on to school or a new career path), one commonality is a loss of identity. If I'm not a tennis player or a gymnast or a swimmer anymore, who am I? For much of their lives, athletes found that their worth was measured in tangible outcomes like wins, losses, points, assists, and times, for example. Everything was measurable, and it's a difficult journey to become comfortable with yourself without that kind of constant external validation.

According to the American Psychiatric Association, preventative measures can help ease the transition for athletes, including the kind of education and awareness opportunities that Meggie suggested, along with help with retirement planning, therapy workshops and support, access to mental health care, and pathways to job training opportunities. And, of course, having broader interests outside of sports, especially during offseason periods when athletes can take on internships, study abroad, or enroll in some classes. One large university in the west has staff members dedicated to study abroad programs where athletes participate in a service project as a group. The same university also helps athletes find internships and supports them in juggling those opportunities with their training and competition schedules. Gaining these meaningful skills and experiences outside of athletics is important, and dedicating staff and resources shows the athletes how to take advantage of everything college can offer.

Leeann, a former soccer player at a mid-Atlantic university, had strongly considered her mental health before she chose a college program. As a talented player who participated in some of the most prestigious and rigorous clubs and camps, she once had visions of going to the Ivy League or D-I level, but after a series of events in high school, her priorities began to shift. She played on the same youth teams as Madison Holleran, a track and field athlete who attended the University of Pennsylvania and died by suicide in her second semester (her story is detailed in the best-selling book *What Made Maddy Run*, by Kate Fagan). The tragedy was a wake-up call to Leeann as she considered her future, having seen a lot of the same traits in herself, like the perfectionism and drive to be the best at everything. Not long afterward, while attending boarding school, Leeann started having a hard time in classes, difficulty waking up in the mornings, and some social anxiety. It was unclear at the time whether she was going through typical teen hormone fluctuations or if she was experiencing symptoms of anxiety. Was a concussion to blame? It may have been a combination of all those factors, but her pediatrician recommended she take anti-anxiety medication, which helped.

Although she wanted to continue playing soccer, she also wanted a situation that allowed her to explore other interests, too, so she chose a D-III school. Unfortunately, the coach of that program was verbally and emotionally abusive, she says—to the point that a group of team members, including Leeann, filed several Title IX complaints for what they felt were persistent microaggressions based on race, gender, sexuality, and socioeconomic status. The complaints were dismissed, but Leeann, once the starting goalkeeper, was cut from the team while she was on an academic trip in Australia, which seemed to her like retaliation. "It was a particularly cruel way to do it," Leeann says. "I called my mom, sobbing. I was confused and angry. It was the worst moment of my life." Her mom encouraged her to get in touch with her therapist. "My therapist said she could pull three years of notes from all of our sessions—all I ever talked about was how terrible this coach made me feel about myself," Leeann says. "From her perspective, I was being let go of something toxic and abusive—and that was the first time she had ever used the word *abusive*. It really hit home for me."

When she arrived back on campus, Leeann started exploring what she could do for her final semesters that might fulfill her in a similar way that soccer always did. During her sophomore year, the women's lacrosse team had been down a few players and they asked her to join. She didn't have a lot of experience in the sport, but it was an opportunity to play for a revered female coach who became an inspiration and role model for how to lead with integrity. It opened Leeann's eyes to the possibility that she, too, might want to pursue the profession. During her final year of college, she opted to play rugby for a club team, where she also encountered a coach (who was male) who also became a valued mentor. Now, Leeann is a high school English teacher and girls' lacrosse coach. "That experience with different coaches taught me that if you build a culture that makes everybody feel valued, nurtured, loved, safe, and like they're part of something special, the winning will come with that," Leeann says. "I'm hard on my girls . . . I hold them accountable and push them hard, but it's coming from a place of love and trust. We've won two championships, but they know if we lose, I'm not going to think any less of them."

REMEMBER YOUR SKILLS

One of the biggest reasons we love sports is because we learn so much that is transferable to so many other aspects of life. And employers love hiring athletes for that very reason. Don't forget that even if you don't know exactly what kind of career you're going to pursue, your participation in sports has already set you up for success by equipping you with the following skills:

- **Setting goals.** You know how to focus on the process to get to the desired outcome.
- **Working hard.** Nobody knows drive and discipline better than an athlete.
- **Leading.** Every player holds a role in keeping the team accountable.
- **Developing teamwork.** You can work with all kinds of other people to achieve a goal.
- **Accepting feedback.** You've spent years making adjustments based on suggestions from coaches.
- **Staying motivated.** You win some, you lose some; you can keep going.
- **Managing time.** You maintained a full course load, a full-time job as an athlete, and still managed to eat, sleep, and get your homework done. The "real world" should seem like a breeze.
- **Thriving under pressure.** Deadlines, presentations, sales pitches. You've got this. You've learned to focus, compete, and perform when it matters most.

FINDING YOURSELF

Not everybody has the ability to immediately seek out help, like Leeann did the night that she was cut from her team. And for many athletes, conflicting and confusing emotions might stop them from looking for support. They've spent a lifetime constantly pushing through hard moments, so why would they change now? But leaving the intensity of athletics is an opportunity to tune into emotional and physical signals that they've been trained to ignore. Athletes also tend to generate heat instead of using cooling rituals to slow down. It's much like the need for physical recovery in training. When you wake up in the morning and your heart rate is elevated, you need to back off for a time to return your nervous system to the parasympathetic state. It's counterintuitive to most athletes' response; they want to forge on instead of slowing down and allowing for recalibration.

Others are embarrassed for feeling such deep grief that their competitive days are over. In the conversations they've had with us, women have consistently acknowledged their privilege: many of them say they enjoyed success in athletics, have great friends, a loving family, and abundant resources. Other people in the world have far worse problems than feeling sad that they are leaving sports, they say. But we also point out, that doesn't mean an athlete shouldn't make space for the hardship, grief, and overwhelm they're experiencing.

Lindsey Richter, a former pro mountain biker, has been through several athletic transitions in her life, ultimately leading to her purpose: getting more women into the sport. Lindsey's relationship with sports started early, dabbling in horseback riding, soccer, basketball, and baseball. She always loved being part of a team, and she enjoyed feeling connected to herself in training. But when she went to college, she decided against pursuing any sports, preferring to immerse herself in classes and socializing. She learned quickly that she had no idea how to function without the structure of practices and competition. Like many athletes who have left organized sports, she had little idea about how to approach exercise merely for the sake of a healthy lifestyle. She tried a little bit of everything, including step aerobics classes, but when nothing stuck, Lindsey fell into depression and an eating disorder. "Learning how to just 'live' without training can be a challenge," she says. "I also think the sense of self can deteriorate without results and instant gratification and cheering."

At age twenty-four, Lindsey discovered mountain bike racing (she also was a cast member on the reality TV show *Survivor* during that time). Although she enjoyed how competition fostered a desire to treat her body better, it was the community, more than anything, that saved her. "The lifestyle of mountain biking helped me heal . . . mountain biking became my therapy," she says. Talk therapy has also helped her understand how to use sport to strengthen her sense of self and realize what she is capable of. In that spirit, she founded Ladies AllRide, a nonprofit organization that teaches women mountain biking skills and how the activity can enhance their lives.

Lindsey says that mountain biking has saved her life—and suggests that retiring athletes try new sports to channel some of the energy and emotions they are coping with, while also starting to build new community connections. "Go into something with a beginner's or growth mindset and find the joy in being new to something," she says. "I think high-performance athletes can isolate themselves sometimes . . . it's important for them to find recreational friends who make it fun."

It's always important to remember that a sport is something you do; it's not who you are. If you haven't gotten the message in each chapter of this book, let us emphasize once again: developing as a whole person—with interests, plans, and friendships that don't hinge solely on your athletic ability—throughout participation in sports is crucial to remaining a healthy and high-performing player and human.

CONCLUSION:
WHY WE HAVE HOPE

How do we improve sports for girls and women?
Start by listening to them.

Abby Wambach said it like this: "One of the things that I feel deeply is when you find something that breaks your heart, turn toward it."

It was at the end of the HBO docuseries[1] showcasing the story of Angel City FC, the National Women's Soccer League expansion team that began playing in 2022. It is founded by three women—actress Natalie Portman, entrepreneur Julie Uhrman, and venture capitalist Kara Nortman—and majority-owned by female investors, including a host of Hollywood and sports celebrities. In the aftermath of the scathing report about systemic abuse, racism, and mistreatment of female soccer players, Abby was referencing the desire to completely change the model and culture of sports for women and girls—who leads them, how we invest in them, and why giving athletes a bigger stake and agency in their own success will improve the outcomes for everybody.

Abby got on board as an investor with Angel City because she believes that all of these changes are possible. And she isn't the only one. "I'm not just going to hear this sad story. I'm going to actually try to figure out what I can do, what I can create, what I can reimagine . . . to fix it."

Angel City FC is founded on the principle that sweeping change is possible not only for women's soccer but for all women's sports—that if you create a profitable and lucrative franchise, set high standards and expectations for the business, players, coaches, and staff, and back it up with a mission that deeply values the athletes, fans, and community, you can elevate the entire league.

Among the first things Angel City's leadership put in place were a code of conduct, reporting mechanisms, and a human resources department—all simple safeguards that were absent in previous iterations of the league, which led to the silencing of athletes who were playing under horrific, abusive circumstances. Angel City team members receive a cut of ticket sales on top of salaries that are starting to better reflect their value. The first player to join Angel City, Christen Press, signed for $700,000 over three years—a far cry from the $5,000 annual salary some players made before the league agreed to a base of $35,000 per year. The club has also created a grant program to help retired players who want to pursue careers in coaching, refereeing, sports media, or the front offices of NWSL teams.

While Angel City's performance on the pitch is a work in progress, its leadership is sticking to the values it's promised to the club and fan base. As a result, it sold an average of nineteen thousand tickets per game in the inaugural season, secured more than $35 million in sponsorships ($1 million of which was reinvested in local organizations that focus on education, food security, sports equity, and LGBTQ+ and gender equality), and saw its club valuation reach more than $100 million, double any other NWSL team. They're proving that it pays to improve working conditions for female athletes and have a clear understanding of your mission.

The deep pockets and enthusiasm of a bunch of famous people have helped move the needle, no doubt. But at its core, Angel City's primary goal is easily replicated. Treat women's sports as a profitable and worthy endeavor on its own, not as an afterthought or second-tier option to men's sports. Provide female athletes the unique care and support that they require as human beings, to perform their best on and off the field. We don't deny that money helps, but the basic premise is not rocket science.

We see a lot of hope in stories like Emily's, the swimmer who began her college career in the Southeast Conference. She emerged from in-patient treatment, thinking she'd never compete again. She wasn't even sure she'd finish her college degree. In time, she realized that she didn't want that experience to define who she was or how she'd finish her collegiate career and landed at a smaller university in the mid-Atlantic with coaches who supported her only stated goal: to finish her competitive swimming career happily.

At her new university, the coaches send out a weekly survey asking about each athlete's academic load that week, what is happening outside of school that might impact training, what their bodies feel like, and how they perceive they are responding to training. After they read the responses, the coaches might pull athletes aside privately and check in on any concerns. It's not a complicated system, but it opens conversations, builds trust, and removes the fear that athletes often experience in talking about their mental health or other problems that impact their athletic performance. And because the coaches consistently follow up, the team knows they care. "I feel reinspired and engaged by a sport I first fell in love with at age seven," Emily says. "I have the most respect for my new coaches because of how much respect they've given me. I feel like I am seen and heard."

AJ is playing basketball in a semipro international league and has found the love of the game again, on a team that supports their identity. It was a meaningful moment when the director of operations asked what pronouns AJ would like used during the play call. To have their identity acknowledged by the system was progress—and today they're helping adolescents as a therapist. "[WNBA player] Layshia [Clarendon] has been a lighthouse for me. Their willingness to be seen as who they are, to advocate for themselves, has granted permission in a way for one reason or another, to do that for myself," AJ says.

Kai, a cross-country runner at a Texas university, became the captain of the campus's chapter of the Hidden Opponent, a national nonprofit organization that raises awareness for student-athlete mental health and addresses the stigma within sports culture. Out of her involvement, she directed five short films for mental health awareness month for the Hidden Opponent's social media channels. At her lowest point in her sophomore year of high school, she was at the mall and noticed posters advertising a major sports apparel brand. Her film, *Win at All Costs?*, highlights the advertising language from sports brands—slogans like "believe in something, even if it means sacrificing everything," against the backdrop of the athletes' reality to expose the fact that our culture prioritizes winning over athlete lives. "We've forgotten that the core of sports isn't about perfection, it's about taking an imperfect human body and doing incredible things with it," Kai says.

That's a recurring theme among all the girls and women we talked with—they're just looking for respect, trust, and to be listened to. We remember that the Women's Sports Foundation research that we covered earlier in this book boiled down to this simple advice for coaching female athletes: "You don't have to be soft, just nice. Do not infantilize or underestimate girls' ability. Treat girls as powerful, strong, very capable individuals." In order to do that, however, we need more clearly defined responsibilities and adequate education for coaches across all sports. They can't continue to function as the last line of defense for everything from training and performance strategies to medical consultant to therapist and nutrition counselor. One person can't provide everything for every athlete, and too often, we are asking coaches to act as experts in areas in which they have no expertise. When they make a mistake simply because they are not provided with the proper resources, it is the athletes who ultimately suffer.

Simultaneously, we need improved systems to hold coaches accountable. Credentialing, mandatory continuing education, and performance metrics beyond win-loss records would all be a great start, weeding out the people who lead with fear tactics, cutthroat mentalities, and disregard their duty to look after the well-being of their athletes as humans with robust identities on and off the field of play.

At the end of our focus groups, we asked a question of our athletes: If you could change one aspect of your athletic career that would have improved your experience, what would you recommend?

"The stigma of mental health would change."

"I'd feel like anybody actually cared."

"Sports psychology would focus on the whole person, not just improving our performance."

"Women would be respected as experts on what they need as athletes."

"Our stories would be celebrated and recognized more."

What we see in this wish list is reflected in various ways in the many stories we told throughout this book, illustrating how female athletes' needs remain unmet in the sports arena. They don't wish for easier training, they don't ask for less pressure in competition, they don't want a less-demanding experience or lower expectations. They want to put their skills on display, test their physical boundaries, and fight as hard as they can for wins within systems that recognize their value, understand and support their needs, and respect their talent, win or lose. It doesn't seem like too much to ask for, does it?

In writing this book, we discovered that what is required of girls and women to show up and compete is more than meets the eye, as we've shown in great detail. They aren't just worried about playing time and scoring points; they're also concerned with how their uniform fits, if they have their period, whether they've convinced enough spectators to show up, and if they look feminine enough (or too feminine or . . . you name it—the body policing never ends). So often, they're coping with misogyny, racism, and mistreatment, too. All these contribute to the mental load these athletes carry from the time they enter sports, and, in turn, their overall mental health.

What would happen if we alleviated those worries and allowed athletes to focus on their performance? Maybe we could make sure they are comfortable in their apparel and put trash cans in the bathroom to throw away their hygiene products. Maybe we could create inclusive environments that embrace all body types. Maybe we could promote their games with the same resources we do the men's competitions, so they can just play. Perhaps we could start by honoring gender and racial identity in sport, too.

Women's sports have come a long way in fifty years, despite operating in the shadows and under a model created specifically for cisgender white men. It's thrilling to imagine what the next fifty years will bring as we continue to pay attention to what female athletes are telling us and changing the game in ways that serve them authentically. Mental health is complex. Many of the best solutions will take time, money, and effort. But starting with basic changes that honor the experiences of thousands of female athletes is a great first step. As Natalie Portman says in the Angel City documentary, "There's no playbook. We have to write our own."

It was a privilege to start here. So many girls and women entrusted their stories to us, hoping that by sharing their experiences, they could improve those of future generations. Their accounts were often painful and personal, but through their vulnerability, their love of sports was also palpable. The magic of athletics lives in all of us, long after we stop playing. They were willing to relive some of their darkest moments because they still believe that sports are worth it—that they can be a place to discover ourselves, defy our perceived limitations, and forge our most meaningful connections.

We'll take Abby's advice and turn toward the heartbreak. In it, we also find hope—and a place to begin again.

EPILOGUE, FROM KATIE

In the winter of 2023, we were in the thick of writing this book. Every day we spoke with athletes from across the country, of all ages, from different sports, and all kinds of athletic backgrounds. And every day we heard these stories—hundreds of them—that were devastating.

During that time, I was skiing up on Mt. Bachelor with my husband, Adam, and I was in a terrible mood. He gently asked me what I needed; I had seemed off for several days, and he could tell I was grappling with something heavy. And at that moment, I burst into tears. The first thing that came out of my mouth was, "These stories are just so sad."

As a clinician, I hear sad stories for a living and I don't think I've ever cried during a session. I care deeply about people, but this was different. Given what I had also been through as an athlete, I am sure I saw flashes of my own experiences in each of the women who shared theirs. Maybe before we started this project, I had believed that conditions for female athletes must have improved, at least a little bit, by now. But my optimism faded as we compiled more anecdotes each day.

A decade after I had left the NCAA, I stepped into a therapist's office and was told I was having an acute trauma response, that my body was holding onto everything I had been through as an athlete, including the years afterward when I still got calls from Alberto and Dr. Brown for blood draws, followed by new prescriptions for altered doses of thyroid medication. My therapist's diagnosis made me scoff, but the truth was, it took that long to feel ready. I had focused on building and nurturing a family and now, with three beautiful kids all growing more independent each day, my bandwidth allowed the floodgates to open.

After that, I dug into everything I could. In the fall of 2021, I took all the medical records I could locate and I spread them out across our living room to create a timeline of a story I thought I knew. I read every word of those records, I talked with doctors who could interpret those documents, and I flew to Arizona to visit with my old coach Marnie to learn exactly why she had left so abruptly during my first year at Oregon. I talked to anybody who might remember anything about those years because, as any therapist will tell you, the brain doesn't like gaps. My body had done its job to protect me: my survival tactic was dissociation, and I didn't remember a lot from my NCAA career. To this day, when anybody discovers that I competed for the University of Oregon track and field team, they are intrigued. When I respond, "I had a pretty hard time in college," it's a real conversation stopper. And that often brings me relief.

Eventually, I moved to EMDR treatment in therapy. In one session, I talked about how alone I felt during college and how I blamed myself for everything that had happened. The therapist held out a stick and told me we'd hold it together. Later, my therapist told me that I pulled hard and tried to hold the stick myself. It was affirmation that I, indeed, have a hard time sharing the burden.

Healing isn't linear, and we can't put fairy-tale endings on any of our stories. I've gotten to a lot of false summits. Sometimes I'm convinced that I'm through the hard parts, but then I find out my doctor needs to change the dosage of my thyroid medication. And I can't do it. I can't force myself to take an extra half of a pill. Nobody gets a clean slate; the trauma is there, but not always *right* there. And it's connected to so many other parts of our lives, too. In the depth of grief for the loss of my dad, who died in 2020 after a long process of early onset Alzheimer's, it connected me with all of my losses and to my process of healing, too. It cracked my whole world wide open, from the inside out, even becoming a catalyst to the conception of this book. While this has been among the most challenging undertakings I've had, it has also proven cathartic. Life presents the time in which we are able to do our work. All our life experiences are linked.

I would not have taken on this project, though, if I didn't feel like we could make meaningful change. I know that sports are worth fighting for. Every athlete who agreed to participate in this book, despite it all, still harbored a deep love for athletics. My hope is that the leaders of leagues, teams, and even the NCAA can understand that what happens under their watch has a long-lasting impact, years after a player moves on. Maybe it gives a few coaches a momentary pause to reflect on how they guide the experiences of their athletes. Is it time to let go of how it's always been done? Discomfort leads to growth.

I don't believe there's anything more powerful than a group of women who are motivated to generate change. At the end of each call with the girls and women who helped us capture the essence of the female athlete experience, each of them said, "Thank you." They were grateful for the opportunity to be brought together, to be valued for their perspective, and to be understood. But most of all, they were thankful to become part of the movement. They volunteered their time and endured grueling conversations because they wanted to help make it better for the next generation. Changemakers, one and all.

Our hope is that in another fifteen years, this book will be obsolete. Female athletes will be developing grit, tenacity, and drive under systems that are made for them, thriving in sports that are inclusive, empowering, and honoring their unique talents. That our collection of stories, however difficult they were to tell, made all the difference.

ATHLETE'S BILL OF RIGHTS

AS AN ATHLETE, YOU HAVE THE RIGHT TO:

1. Be treated with respect and dignity by coaches, staff, teammates, spectators, and fans.
2. Train and compete in a safe environment, free from exploitation, abuse, bullying, belittling, physical harm, harassment, violence, or threats from coaches, staff, or teammates.
3. Participate, regardless of your identity, as well as receive affirmation of your identity.
4. Be understood as a whole person, who has many distinct interests, activities, concerns, and identities separate from sports.
5. Mental health support and treatment that is as easily accessible as physical support and treatment and gives you a voice in decisions that involve your mental health care.
6. Transparency regarding team policies and procedures that are fair, free from favoritism and conflicts of interest, and allow you to report improper behavior or violations of SafeSport code without fear of retribution.
7. Inclusion and support during recovery from illness, injury, and other setbacks.
8. Adequate time for basic needs like nutrition, sleep, and recovery.
9. Privacy concerning your mental health needs, free from worry that coaches and staff might share your information without your permission.
10. Coaching that is representative, qualified, compassionate, and takes your input and concerns into account.

GRATITUDE

We are beyond lucky to have such a long list of people to thank for their immeasurable contributions. Whether you jumped on a phone call, answered an early morning text, or shared your thoughts with us, *The Price She Pays* would not be what it is without your love.

Thank you, Susan Canavan and Waxman Literary Agency. You believed in us and this project before it was even fully hatched. We appreciate that you took a leap with two therapists—and in doing so, you became our North Star and fiercest advocate throughout the entire process.

Thank you, Erin Strout, for your literary acumen. You are an absolute word wizard, brilliant human, and a saint for partnering with two clinicians who are process-driven and learning a whole new industry. It's been the delight of a lifetime getting to work with you and to know you. You left us wonderstruck on a regular basis, and we admire you evermore. You are a champion of women in ways this book deserved.

Thank you to our editors Talia Krohn, Marisa Vigilante, and the Little, Brown Spark team for your leadership, expertise, and wisdom. From our first meeting, the connection and passion we all shared for athletes' mental health was palpable.

Thank you, Chris Roslan, of Roslan and Associates Public Relations, for your eagerness to advocate for the mental health of athletes. Your immediate belief in us elevated our purpose.

A heartfelt thank you to The Hidden Opponent, who generously and quickly connected us with athletes who comprised some of our most influential focus groups. The work you are doing is changing the world for athletes and mental health.

To the kids in our lives—we hope this work leads to better athletic systems for your futures. Thank you for continuously showing us how to embody joy, humor, and fun in every situation. Watching you stay true to yourselves makes us the most proud. You are the real change agents, no matter your path, and we will always be advocating and rooting for you.

We extend appreciation to our dearest friends and family who helped us navigate a world of writing we knew nothing about. Cheers to your boundless support and (albeit ridiculous) belief in our dream. We are deeply grateful you are our people.

We have the luxury of working with incredible people who nurtured us in this process. It is a gift to learn beside you and to mutually cultivate continual growth—professionally, academically, and clinically. The work you do, with unlimited compassion to support our communities, is relentlessly inspiring.

To all the students and clients we have had the opportunity to know over the years—working with you is the ultimate privilege.

And, finally, this book is a collective effort. To everyone who shared their time and experiences with us, saying thank you seems inadequate. We are deeply grateful that you trusted us to steward your stories. We appreciate how you opened up your worlds and voiced your most vulnerable truths. We admire you endlessly.

ADDITIONAL RESOURCES

A select list of organizations and other sources
of information and support.

ABUSE, MISTREATMENT, AND TRAUMA

The Army of Survivors

Thearmyofsurvivors.org

Bringing awareness, accountability, and transparency to sexual violence against athletes at all levels, created by survivors of sexual assault in USA Gymnastics.

RAINN

Rainn.org

Rape, Abuse & Incest National Network (RAINN) is the nation's largest anti-sexual violence organization. RAINN also carries out programs to prevent sexual violence, help survivors, and ensure that perpetrators are brought to justice.

The US Center for SafeSport

Uscenterforsafesport.org

An independent nonprofit organization working toward a sport community free of emotional, physical, and sexual abuse and misconduct, providing training resources and best practices for coaches, parents, athletes, youth, and amateur sports. Receives and responds to allegations of abuse and misconduct in sport through a confidential online form or by phone at 833-5US-SAFE.

ATHLETE MENTAL HEALTH SUPPORT

Athletes Mental Health Foundation
Athletesmentalhealthfoundation.org
A nonprofit organization dedicated to helping athletes understand and address their internal well-being and optimizes the integration of mental health in athletic systems. Aimed at helping athletes perform better and find more love for their sports through enhanced mental wellness.

The Hidden Opponent
Thehiddenopponent.org
An advocacy group that raises awareness for student-athlete mental health and addresses the stigma within sports culture. The community is a safe space for all student-athletes to feel heard, supported, and loved, providing free access and support from mental health professionals and experts in the field.

Katie's Save
Katiessave.org
A nonprofit organization advocating to implement a policy in which students can opt for a trusted adult "designated advocate" to receive notice and provide support when they need it most.

Morgan's Message
Morgansmessage.org
A nonprofit organization that strives to eliminate the stigma surrounding mental health within the student-athlete community and equalize the treatment of physical and mental health in athletics, aiming to expand the dialogue on mental health by normalizing conversations, empowering those who suffer in silence, and supporting those who feel alone.

National Alliance on Mental Illness

Nami.org

The nation's largest grassroots mental health organization dedicated to building better lives for the millions of Americans affected by mental illness.

National Suicide & Crisis Lifeline

988lifeline.org

Provides free and confidential emotional support to people in suicidal crisis or emotional distress twenty-four-hours-a-day, seven-days-a-week in the United States. If you are thinking about harming yourself or attempting suicide, call 988.

BODY IMAGE AND EATING DISORDERS

The Emily Program

Emilyprogram.com

Nationally recognized for eating disorder awareness and treatment, whose mission is to provide individualized care leading to recovery.

Families Empowered and Supporting Treatment for Eating Disorders (FEAST)

Feast-ed.org

An international organization of and for caregivers of loved ones suffering from eating disorders, providing information and mutual support, promoting evidence-based treatment, and advocating for research and education to reduce the suffering associated with eating disorders.

National Eating Disorder Association

Nationaleatingdisorders.org

The largest nonprofit organization dedicated to supporting individuals and families affected by eating disorders, serving as a catalyst for prevention, cures, and access to quality care.

Project Heal

Theprojectheal.org

Their mission is to break down systemic, health care, and financial barriers to eating disorder healing with a multitude of programs to provide lifesaving support to people with eating disorders to whom the system fails.

RED in Sport

Redinsport.org

A site about Relative Energy Deficiency in Sports, updated by professionals in the fields of sports medicine treatment and research who believe every athlete, coach, parent, trainer, and supporter should be aware of the risks posed by underfueling, as well as how to avoid and identify these risks.

Running in Silence

Runninginsilence.org

Empowering the athletic community through eating disorder education and awareness so athletes can receive help and achieve their potential in health and athletic performance.

GIRLS' AND WOMEN'S HEALTH

Black Women's Health Imperative

Bwhi.org

Solely dedicated to achieving health equity for Black women in America. BWHI has evolved into a nationally recognized organization leading health policy, education, research, knowledge, and leadership development and communications designed to improve the healthy outcomes of Black women.

Bras for Girls

Brasforgirls.org

Donates new, high-quality sports bras and breast-development education booklets to girls in need, ages eight to eighteen. Recipient programs include sports teams, school programs, community programs, and other initiatives that elevate girls' access to sports.

Sex Positive Families

Sexpositivefamilies.com

Provides education and resources that help families raise sexually healthy children using a shame-free and comprehensive approach.

Stanford FASTR Program

Fastr.stanford.edu

Seeking to better understand the female athlete and provide the resources to make optimal health and performance more accessible to female athletes of all ages and skill levels.

Vaughn Childcare Fund

Vaughnchildcarefund.org

Providing funds for childcare to parenting student athletes, as well as information, education, and mentoring.

Wu Tsai Female Athlete Program at Boston Children's Hospital

Childrenshospital.org

Taking a comprehensive approach to diagnosing, treating, and managing sports injuries in female athletes by assessing the whole athlete, including exercise habits, hormonal balance, and nutritional needs—not just symptoms and injuries—to ensure peak performance.

HUMAN RIGHTS AND SOCIAL JUSTICE

Athlete Ally

Athleteally.org

The Athlete Ally mission is to end homophobia and transphobia in sport and to activate the athletic community to exercise its leadership to champion LGBTQI+ equality.

Black Women in Sport Foundation

Blackwomeninsport.org

A nonprofit organization whose mission is to increase the involvement of Black women and girls in all aspects of sport, including athletics, coaching, and administration.

InterACT

Interactadvocates.org

InterACT's mission is to use innovative legal and other strategies to advocate for the human rights of children born with intersex traits, including athletics.

Mom of All Capes

Momofallcapes.com

Elevating diverse voices and perspectives in the civic education space, working with students, educators, and parent communities for more equitable outcomes.

NCAA Gender Equity and Title IX Information

NCAA.org

Information about federal and state laws regarding gender equity.

TransAthlete.com, by Chris Mosier

Transathlete.com

An evolving resource for students, athletes, coaches, and administrators to find information about trans inclusion in athletics at various levels of play.

The Trevor Project

Thetrevorproject.org

The Trevor Project's mission is to end suicide among LGTBQ young people through crisis support, advocacy, research, and education.

SUBSTANCE USE

Alcoholics Anonymous
Aa.org
Alcoholics Anonymous provides free information, mutual aid, and resources to support anyone seeking to stop using substances.

Association of Recovery in Higher Education
Collegiaterecovery.org
ARHE provides the education, resources, and community connection needed to help change the trajectory of recovering students' lives.

National Harm Reduction Coalition
Harmreduction.org
The National Harm Reduction Coalition creates spaces for dialogue and action that help heal the harm caused by racialized drug policies. Its work is aimed to create, sustain, and expand evidence-based harm reduction programs and policies.

Refuge Recovery
Refugerecovery.org
Refuge Recovery, based on Buddhist principles, provides tools and support for healing with substance use and the suffering induced by substance use.

Sober Black Girls Club
Soberblackgirlsclub.com
This collective provides resources and support to Black girls, women, femmes, and nonbinary folks practicing sobriety, in recovery, or considering it.

Substance Abuse and Mental Health Services Administration (SAMHSA)

Samhsa.gov

SAMHSA is the agency within the US Department of Health and Human Services that leads public health efforts to advance the behavioral health of the nation.

White Bison

Whitebison.org

White Bison provides sobriety, recovery, prevention, and wellness/Wellbriety learning resources to the Native American/Alaskan Native community nationwide.

SUICIDE AND SELF-HARM

988 Suicide and Crisis Lifeline

988lifeline.org

The 988 Lifeline is a national network of local crisis centers that provides free and confidential emotional support to people in suicidal crisis or emotional distress twenty-four hours a day, seven days a week in the United States. Call 988 from any phone.

Cornell Research Program on Self-Injury

Selfinjury.bctr.cornell.edu

Dedicated to sharing resources related to self-injury and associated conditions and translating the growing body of knowledge about self-injury into resources and tools.

Crisis Text Line

Crisistextline.org

A national nonprofit that provides a significant number of resources for a variety of mental health needs. Includes a 24/7 text line for anyone in crisis. Text HOME to 741741 from anywhere in the United States. A trained crisis counselor receives the text and responds from a secure online platform.

To Write Love on Her Arms

Twloha.com

A nonprofit movement dedicated to presenting hope and finding help for people struggling with depression, addiction, self-injury, and suicide; aimed to encourage, inform, inspire, and invest directly into treatment and recovery.

WOMEN'S SPORTS ADVOCACY

&Mother

Andmother.org

Advocating for a healthy and productive society where everyone prospers because of the contributions of women and mothers; where the value of mothers in the workforce is intrinsic, and motherhood is not a limiting factor in how women succeed professionally and personally.

Play It Forward Sport

Playitforwardsport.org

Aims to advance gender equality by creating opportunities and sharing the inspiration of women's sports by empowering female athletes to play forward their talents and experiences as they inspire, educate, and mentor others to reach their dreams.

The Tucker Center for Girls and Women in Sports

Cehd.umn.edu/tuckercenter

An interdisciplinary research center at the University of Minnesota leading a global effort to accelerate change for girls and women in sport and physical activity and their families and communities. Experts conduct solution-based research, translate knowledge, provide educational opportunities, and engage in community outreach that impact girls and women in sport and physical activity.

Women Leadership in Sports

Womenleadersinsports.org

Women Leaders is an expanding membership community of women and men who strive to grow as leaders and believe in diversity and equity in leadership.

Women's Sports Foundation

Womenssportsfoundation.org

Through research, advocacy, community impact, and partnerships, the foundation is building a future where every girl and woman can play, be active, and realize her full potential.

YOUTH SPORTS

American Academy of Pediatrics

Aap.org

The academy of sixty-seven thousand pediatricians committed to the optimal physical, mental, and social health and well-being for all infants, children, adolescents, and young adults.

Center for Healing and Justice through Sport

Chjs.org

The CHJS was created to use sport as an intentional strategy to support healing, build resilience, and address issues of systemic injustice. The group considers the ways sport is uniquely situated to help kids heal and thrive.

Go Z Girls

zgirls.org

Teaching girls the mental skills needed to overcome self-doubt and build lifelong confidence through online programs with professional and Olympic female athletes.

National Council of Youth Sports

Ncys.org

NCYS is an advocate for young people to have full access to sports and to ensure that games are played in safe environments.

Project Play, an Initiative of the Aspen Institute's Sports & Society Program

Projectplay.org

Project Play develops, applies, and shares knowledge that helps build healthy communities through sports.

TrueSport

Truesport.org

TrueSport is an initiative of the US Anti-Doping Agency, with a mission to change the culture of youth sport by providing educational tools to equip young athletes with the resources to build life skills and core values for success on and off the field. Educational programs and coaching certifications are available through TrueSport.

NOTES

INTRODUCTION

1   "Vin Lananna," GoDucks, University of Oregon, https://goducks.com
/sports/track-and-field/roster/coaches/vin-lananna/241.

2   "AAA Panel Imposes 4-Year Sanctions on Alberto Salazar and Dr. Jeffrey
Brown for Multiple Anti-Doping Rules Violations," United States Anti-
Doping Agency, September 30, 2019, https://www.usada.org/sanction/aaa
-panel-4-year-sanctions-alberto-salazar-jeffrey-brown/.

3   Mary Cain, "I Was the Fastest Girl in America, until I Joined Nike," *New
York Times*, November 7, 2019, https://www.nytimes.com/2019/11/07
/opinion/nike-running-mary-cain.html.

4   Kara Goucher, *The Longest Race: Inside the Secret World of Abuse, Doping, and
Deception on Nike's Elite Running Team* (New York: Gallery Books, 2023).

5   Mike Penner, "U.S. Gymnast Braves Pain for Gold," *Los Angeles Times*, July
24, 1996.

CHAPTER 1

1   "U.S. Olympic & Paralympic Committee Announces 613-Member 2020
U.S. Olympic Team," Team USA, July 13, 2021, https://www.teamusa
.com/news/2021/july/13/usopc-announces-613-member-2020-us
-olympic-team.

2   "From the Shadows to the Spotlight," Wasserman and ESPNW Research,
October 2023, https://www.teamwass.com/news/new-study-womens
-sports-comprise-15-of-sports-media-coverage/.

3   J. Glaaser, C. Boucher, and N. M. LaVoi, "A New Era. The Women in
College Coaching Report Card, Year 11: Select Seven NCAA Division-I
institutions, 2022–23," The Tucker Center for Research on Girls &

Women in Sport, August 2023, https://wecoachsports.org/wp-content
/uploads/WCCRC-SELECT-SEVEN-2023_August-1-2023.pdf.

4   "The American College of Sports Medicine Statement on Mental Health
    Challenges for Athletes," American College of Sports Medicine, August 9,
    2021, https://www.acsm.org/news-detail/2021/08/09/the-american
    -college-of-sports-medicine-statement-on-mental-health-challenges-for
    -athletes.

5   "The State of Mental Health in America," Mental Health America. Accessed
    December 27, 2023, https://mhanational.org/issues/state-mental-health
    -america.

6   Ernst & Young, "Where Will You Find Your Next Leader?" Accessed
    March 26, 2024, https://www.ey.com/en_us/athlete-programs/why
    -female-athletes-should-be-your-next-leader.

CHAPTER 2

1   Kelsey Logan et al., "Organized Sports for Children, Preadolescents, and
    Adolescents," *Pediatrics* 143, no. 6 (June 2019): e20190997. https://doi
    .org/10.1542/peds.2019-0997.

2   "State of Play 2022," The Aspen Institute. Accessed December 27, 2023,
    https://projectplay.org/state-of-play-2022/costs-to-play-trends.

3   "State of Play 2019," The Aspen Institute. Accessed December 27, 2023,
    https://www.aspeninstitute.org/wp-content/uploads/2019/10/2019_SOP
    _National_Final.pdf.

4   "Do You Know What's Influencing Girls' Participation in Sports?" The
    Women's Sports Foundation. Accessed December 27, 2023, https://www
    .womenssportsfoundation.org/do-you-know-the-factors-influencing-girls
    -participation-in-sports/.

5   J. L. Herman, A. R. Flores, and K. K. O'Neill, "How Many Adults and Youth
    Identify as Transgender in the United States?" The Williams Institute, UCLA
    School of Law. Accessed December 27, 2023, https://williamsinstitute.law.
    ucla.edu/wp-content/uploads/Trans-Pop-Update-Jun-2022.pdf.

6   "The Trevor Project Research Brief: LGBTQ Youth Sports Participation,"
    The Trevor Project, September 2021, https://www.thetrevorproject.org/wp
    -content/uploads/2021/09/LGBTQ-Youth-and-Sports_-September
    -Research-Brief-2.pdf.

7   Sally Yates, "Report of the Independent Investigation to the U.S. Soccer
    Federation Concerning Allegations of Abusive Behavior and Sexual

Misconduct in Women's Professional Soccer," King & Spalding, October 3, 2022, https://www.kslaw.com/attachments/000/009/931/original/King ___Spalding_-_Full_Report_to_USSF.pdf?1664809048.

CHAPTER 3

1   "Estimated Probability of Competing in NCAA Athletics," NCAA. Accessed December 27, 2023, https://www.ncaa.org/sports/2015/3/2 /estimated-probability-of-competing-in-college-athletics.aspx.

2   Tressie McMillan Cottom, "Venus and Serena Williams on Their Own Terms," *Harper's Bazaar,* February 16, 2022, https://www.harpersbazaar .com/culture/features/a38957619/0001-0179-origin-story-march-2022/.

CHAPTER 4

1   "Coach Well-Being Survey," NCAA, January 26, 2023, https://ncaaorg .s3.amazonaws.com/research/wellness/2023RES_NCAA-Coach-Well -BeingSurveyReport.pdf.

2   R. Hughes and J. Coakley, "Positive Deviance among Athletes: The Implications of Overconformity to the Sport Ethic," *Sociology of Sport Journal* 8, no. 4 (1991): 307–25, https://doi.org/10.1123/ssj.8.4.307.

3   N. Zarrett, C. Cooky, and P. T. Veliz, "Coaching through a Gender Lens: Maximizing Girls' Play and Potential," Women's Sports Foundation, April 2, 2019. https://www.womenssportsfoundation.org/wp-content/uploads /2019/04/coaching-through-a-gender-lens-report-web.pdf

4   "State of Play 2022," The Aspen Institute. Accessed December 27, 2023, https://projectplay.org/state-of-play-2022/coaching-trends.

5   "Quality Coaching Framework," US Olympic and Paralympic Committee. Accessed December 28, 2023, https://www.usopc.org/quality-coaching -framework.

6   Glaaser, Boucher, and LaVoi, "A New Era." https://www.cehd.umn.edu /tuckercenter/library/docs/research/WCCRC-2022-23-Select-7.pdf

7   Zarrett, Cooky, and Veliz, "Coaching through a Gender Lens." https:// www.womenssportsfoundation.org/wp-content/uploads/2019/04/coaching -through-a-gender-lens-report-web.pdf

8   "A Look at Trends for Women in College Sports," NCAA, March 1, 2023, https://www.ncaa.org/news/2023/3/1/media-center-a-look-at-trends-for -women-in-college-sports.aspx.

CHAPTER 5

1   "Physical Changes during Puberty," American Academy of Pediatrics. Accessed December 28, 2023, https://www.healthychildren.org/English /ages-stages/gradeschool/puberty/Pages/Physical-Development-of-School -Age-Children.aspx.

2   Maham Javaid, "After a 1935 Tragedy, a Priest Vowed to Teach Kids about Menstruation," *Washington Post,* March 25, 2023, https://www.washington post.com/nation/2023/03/25/florida-schools-bill-menstruation-crisis -suicide-hotline-mcclain/.

3   Lauren Fleshman, "Dear Younger Me," Milesplit USA. Accessed December 28, 2017, https://www.milesplit.com/articles/211759/dear-younger-me -lauren-fleshman.

4   Erin Strout, "Orlando Pride Is Ditching Its White Shorts So Players Are Never Uncomfortable on Their Periods," *Women's Health,* February 28, 2023, https://www.womenshealthmag.com/fitness/a43104333/orlando -pride-updates-uniform-look-periods/.

5   J. Scurr, N. Brown, J. Smith, A. Brasher, D. Risius, and A. Marczyk, "The Influence of the Breast on Sport and Exercise Participation in School Girls in the United Kingdom" *Journal of Adolescent Health* 58, no. 2 (February 2016):167–73, doi:10.1016/j.jadohealth.2015.10.005.

CHAPTER 6

1   J. C. Basso and W. A. Suzuki, "The Effects of Acute Exercise on Mood, Cognition, Neurophysiology, and Neurochemical Pathways: A Review," *Brain Plasticity* 2, no. 2, (March 28, 2017): 127–52. doi: 10.3233/BPL -160040.

2   C. P. Herrero, N. Jejurikar, and C. W. Carter, "The Psychology of the Female Athlete: How Mental Health and Wellness Mediate Sports Performance, Injury and Recovery," *Annals of Joint* 6 (2021): 38.

3   *Diagnostic and Statistical Manual of Mental Disorders* (Washington, DC: American Psychiatric Association Publishers, 2022).

4   Herrero, Jejurikar, and Carter, "The Psychology of the Female Athlete."

5   "Simone Manuel Gives Emotional Press Conference Explaining Overtraining Syndrome Diagnosis," SwimSwam, June 18, 2021, https:// www.youtube.com/watch?v=hJ8BVYmRrek.

6   "Simone Manuel's Journey Back to Swimming since the Tokyo Olympics,"
     SwimSwam, March 28, 2023, https://swimswam.com/simone-manuels
     -journey-back-to-swimming-since-the-tokyo-olympics/.

CHAPTER 7

1   Simone Biles, "Statement for 9/15 Hearing," US Senate Committee on
     the Judiciary, November 15, 2021, https://www.judiciary.senate.gov/imo
     /media/doc/Biles%20Testimony1.pdf.
2   Marisa Kwiatkowski, Mark Alesia, and Tim Evans, "A Blind Eye to Sex
     Abuse: How USA Gymnastics Failed to Report Cases," *Indianapolis Star,*
     August 4, 2016, https://www.indystar.com/story/news/investigations
     /2016/08/04/usa-gymnastics-sex-abuse-protected-coaches/85829732/.
3   "Sparking Cultural Change for a Safer Tomorrow: U.S. Center for
     SafeSport 2022 Annual Report," US Center for SafeSport, 2022. Accessed
     December 28, 2023,https://uscenterforsafesport.org/2022-annual-report/.
4   Aly Raisman, "Statement to the U.S. Senate Committee on the Judiciary,"
     September 15, 2021, https://www.judiciary.senate.gov/imo/media/doc
     /Raisman%20Testimony.pdf.
5   "2020 Athlete Culture & Climate Survey," US Center for SafeSport, July
     14, 2021, https://uscenterforsafesport.org/wp-content/uploads/2021/07
     /CultureClimateSurvey_ExternalReport_071421_Final.pdf.
6   Shelba Waldron, "Tough Coaching or Emotional Abuse: Knowing When
     the Line Has Been Crossed," USA Gymnastics SafeSport Training. Accessed
     December 28, 2023, https://members.usagym.org/PDFs/Member%20
     Services/webinars/ss_emotional.pdf.
7   Dale Vernor, "PTSD Is More Likely in Women Than Men," National
     Alliance on Mental Illness, October 8, 2019, https://www.nami.org
     /Blogs/NAMI-Blog/October-2019/PTSD-is-More-Likely-in-Women
     -Than-Men.
8   A. L. Roberts, M. Rosario, H. L. Corliss, K. C. Koenen, and S. B. Austin,
     "Elevated Risk of Post-Traumatic Stress in Sexual Minority Youths:
     Mediation by Childhood Abuse and Gender Nonconformity," *American
     Journal of Public Health* 102, no. 8. (August 2012): 1587–93. doi:10.2105
     /AJPH.2011.300530.
9   Natalie Guitiérrez, *The Pain We Carry: Healing from Complex PTSD for
     People of Color* (Oakland, CA: New Harbinger Publications, 2022).

NOTES

10 Judith Herman, *Trauma and Recovery: The Aftermath of Violence—From Domestic Abuse to Political Terror,* (New York: Basic Books, 1992).

11 Bob Hohler, "A Reckoning, Decades in the Making: Famed Olympic Runner Lynn Jennings Chases Down the Renowned Coach Who Abused Her as a Teen," *Boston Globe,* February 17, 2023, https://www.bostonglobe.com/2023/02/17/sports/lynn-jennings-john-babington/.

12 "Boston Globe Story on Sexual Abuse Perpetrated by Former Wellesley College Coach John Babington," Wellesley, February 17, 2023, https://blogs.wellesley.edu/announcements/2023/02/17/boston-globe-story-on-sexual-abuse-perpetrated-by-former-wellesley-coach-john-babington/.

13 Molly Hensley-Clancy, "Nobody Cares: NWSL Players Say U.S. Soccer Failed to Act on Abuse Claims Against Red Stars Coach," *Washington Post,* November 22, 2021, https://www.washingtonpost.com/sports/2021/11/22/rory-dames-chicago-red-stars-resigns/.

14 Meg Linehan, "'This Guy Has a Pattern': Amid Institutional Failure, Former NWSL Players Accuse Prominent Coach of Sexual Coercion," *The Athletic,* September 30, 2021, https://theathletic.com/2857633/2021/09/30/this-guy-has-a-pattern-amid-institutional-failure-former-nwsl-players-accuse-prominent-coach-of-sexual-coercion/.

15 Scott Reid, "Attorney Alleges UC Berkeley Coach Teri McKeever is the Victim of Gender Bias," *OC Register,* June 25, 2022, https://www.ocregister.com/2022/06/25/attorney-alleges-uc-berkeley-coach-teri-mckeever-is-the-victim-of-gender-bias/.

CHAPTER 8

1 Matthew Futterman, "Jessie Diggins Wins Bronze in Individual Sprint, Her Second Olympic Medal," *New York Times,* February 8, 2022, https://www.nytimes.com/2022/02/07/sports/olympics/jessie-diggins-bronze-sprint-cross-country.html.

2 Jessie Diggins (@jessiediggins), "Working on a blog post about the Games that I might (someday) finish," Instagram photo, March 7, 2022, https://www.instagram.com/p/Ca0HRC3uO35/?utm_source=ig_web_copy_link.

3 Jessie Diggins, "Body Issue(s)," *Jessie Diggins* (blog), June 25, 2018, https://jessiediggins.com/body-issues/.

4 S. Bratland-Sanda and J. Sundgot-Borgen, "Eating Disorders in Athletes: Overview of Prevalence, Risk Factors and Recommendations for

258

Prevention and Treatment," *European Journal of Sport Science* 13, no. 5 (2013): 499–508. doi:10.1080/17461391.2012.740504. Accessed December 28, 2023.

5   K. Kato, S. Jevas, and D. Culpepper, "Body Image Disturbances in NCAA Division I and III Female Athletes," *The Sport Journal,* https://thesport journal.org/article/body-image-disturbances-in-ncaa-division-i-and-iii -female-athletes/.

6   Deloitte Access Economics. "The Social and Economic Cost of Eating Disorders in the United States of America: A Report for the Strategic Training Initiative for the Prevention of Eating Disorders and the Academy for Eating Disorders," Harvard School of Public Health, June 2020, https://www.hsph.harvard.edu/striped/report-economic-costs-of-eating -disorders/.

7   Ken Goe, "Women Athletes Allege Body Shaming within Oregon Ducks Track and Field Program," *The Oregonian,* October 25, 2021, https://www .oregonlive.com/trackandfield/2021/10/women-athletes-allege-body -shaming-within-oregon-ducks-track-and-field-program.html.

CHAPTER 9

1   Steven Meyer and Gina Meyer, Individually and as Successor in Interest to Kathryn Diane Meyer vs. The Leland Stanford Junior University, et al., 22CV407844 (Superior Court of California County of Santa Clara, 2022).

2   A. L. Rao, I. M. Asif, J. A. Drezner, B. G. Toresdahl, and K. G. Harmon, "Suicide in National Collegiate Athletic Association (NCAA) Athletes: A 9-Year Analysis of the NCAA Resolutions Database," *Sports Health* 7, no. 5 (September–October 2015): 452–57. doi:10.1177/1941738115587675.

3   D. M. Stone, K. A. Mack, and J. Qualters, "*Notes from the Field:* Recent Changes in Suicide Rates, by Race and Ethnicity and Age Group—United States, 2021," *Morbidity and Mortality Weekly Report* 72 (2023): 160–62. http://dx.doi.org/10.15585/mmwr.mm7206a4.

4   "The Youth Risk Behavior Survey," Centers for Disease Control and Prevention, 2011–2021. Accessed December 28, 2023, https://www.cdc .gov/healthyyouth/data/yrbs/yrbs_data_summary_and_trends.htm?s_cid =hy-DSTR1-2023.

5   Amy E. Green, Jonah P. DeChants, Myeshia N. Price, and Carrie K. Davis, "Association of Gender-Affirming Hormone Therapy with Depression,

Thoughts of Suicide, and Attempted Suicide among Transgender and Nonbinary Youth," *Journal of Adolescent Health* 70, no. 4 (December 14, 2021), https://doi.org/10.1016/j.jadohealth.2021.10.036.

CHAPTER 10

1 "188. Abby Wambach: Will I Ever Be Truly Loved?" March 2023, in *We Can Do Hard Things*, podcast, MP3 audio, hosted by Abby Wambach, Glennon Doyle, and Amanda Doyle, https://podcasts.apple.com/us /podcast/188-abby-wambach-will-i-ever-be-truly-loved/id1564530722?i =1000604046032.

2 Abby Wambach, *Forward: A Memoir* (Dey Street Books, New York, 2017).

3 Hannah B. Apsley, Noel Vest, Kyler S. Knapp, Alexis Santos-Lozada, Joy Gray, Gregory Hard, and Abenaa A. Jones, "Non-Engagement in Substance Use Treatment among Women with an Unmet Need for Treatment: A Latent Class Analysis on Multidimensional Barriers," *Drug and Alcohol Dependence* 242 (January 2023): 109715, https://doi.org/10.1016/j.drug alcdep.2022.109715.

4 "2021 National Survey on Drug Use and Health," Substance Abuse and Mental Health Services Administration, 2021. Accessed December 28, 2023, https://www.samhsa.gov/data/release/2021-national-survey-drug -use-and-health-nsduh-releases.

5 "2017 NCAA Student-Athlete Substance Use Survey," NCAA, 2017, https://www.ncaa.org/sports/2013/11/20/ncaa-student-athlete-substance -use-study.aspx.

6 H. H. Cleveland, K. S. Harris, A. K. Baker, R. Herbert, and L. R. Dean, "Characteristics of a Collegiate Recovery Community: Maintaining Recovery in an Abstinence-Hostile Environment," *Journal of Substance Abuse Treatment* 33, no. 1, (July 2007): 13–23. doi:10.1016/j.jsat.2006 .11.005.

7 Brian Hainline, Lydia Bell, and Mary Wilfert, "Mind, Body, Sport: Substance Use and Abuse," NCAA, https://www.ncaa.org/sports/2014 /11/4/mind-body-and-sport-substance-use-and-abuse.aspx.

8 Michelle Pitts, Graig Chow, and Yang Yanyun, "Athletes' Perceptions of Their Head Coach's Alcohol Management Strategies and Athlete Alcohol Use," *Addiction Research & Theory* 26 (2017): 1–9. doi:10.1080/16066359 .2017.1341976.

9   Kevin McCauley, https://drkevinmccauley.com/.

10   "Delaware State Agencies Partner with Youth Sports Team to Prevent
      Opioid Use," February 9, 2023, https://news.delaware.gov/2023/02/09
      /delaware-state-agencies-partner-with-youth-sports-teams-to-prevent
      -opioid-use-among-teen-athletes/.

CHAPTER 11

1   Alexis, Kathleen, and Jeffrey Spence vs. Meta Platforms Inc., 3:22-cv-
      03294 (United States District Court Northern District of California San
      Francisco Division, June 6, 2022), https://socialmediavictims.org/wp
      -content/uploads/2022/06/Spence-Complaint-6_6_22.pdf.

2   Cristiano Lima, "A Whistleblower's Power: Key Takeaways from the
      Facebook Papers," *Washington Post,* October 26, 2021, https://www
      .washingtonpost.com/technology/2021/10/25/what-are-the-facebook
      -papers/.

3   Simone Biles (@Simone_Biles), "you all can judge my body all you want,
      but at the end of the day it's MY body. I love it & I'm comfortable in my
      skin," X (formerly Twitter), December 27, 2016, https://twitter.com
      /Simone_Biles/status/813947733816016896.

4   Ben Rothenberg, "Tennis's Top Women Balance Body Image with
      Ambition," *New York Times,* July 10, 2015, https://www.nytimes.com
      /2015/07/11/sports/tennis/tenniss-top-women-balance-body-image-with
      -quest-for-success.html.

5   Kareem Abdul-Jabbar, "Body Shaming Black Female Athletes Is Not Just
      about Race," *Newsweek,* July 20, 2015, https://time.com/3964758/body
      -shaming-black-female-athletes/.

6   "World Athletics Publishes Abuse Study Covering Tokyo Olympic Games,"
      World Athletics, November 25, 2021, https://worldathletics.org/news
      /press-releases/online-abuse-study-athletes-tokyo-olympic-games.

7   "World Athletics Publishes Online Abuse Study Covering World Athletic
      Championships Oregon22," World Athletics, December 2, 2022, https://
      worldathletics.org/news/press-releases/online-abuse-study-world-athletics
      -championships-oregon22.

8   Evelyn Watta, "British Pole Vaulter Holly Bradshaw Scarred by Online
      Abuse," Olympics.com, March 22, 2023, https://olympics.com/en/news
      /british-pole-vaulter-holly-bradshaw-online-abuse.

9   Sedona Price (@sedonerr), "it's 2021 and we are still fighting for bits and pieces of equality. #ncaa #inequality #fightforchange," TikTok post, March 18, 2022, https://www.tiktok.com/@sedonerrr/video/6941180 880127888646.

10   "Kaplan Hecker & Fink Releases Independent Review and Recommendations around Gender Issues in NCAA Championships," Kaplan Hecker & Fink LLP, August 3, 2021, https://ncaagenderequity review.com/phase-i-report-announcement/.

11   ESPN (@espn), "9.9 MILLION VIEWERS Record-breaking #NationalChampionship thriller between @LSUwbkb and @IowaWBB makes TV history," X (formerly Twitter) post, April 3, 2023, https://x.com /ESPNPR/status/1643004893655965706?s=20.

12   Remy Tumin, "NCAA Women's Tournament Shatters Ratings Record in Final," *New York Times*, April 3, 2023, https://www.nytimes.com/2023 /04/03/sports/ncaabasketball/lsu-iowa-womens-tournament-ratings-record .html.

13   "Angel Reese," On3 NIL Deals, https://www.on3.com/db/angel-reese -174581/nil-deals/.

14   NBC Sports Washington Staff, "WNBA Salaries, Who Has the Highest, League Average, and More," Yahoo Sports, May 31, 2023, https://sports .yahoo.com/wnba-salaries-highest-league-average-140000974.html.

15   "Emily Cole," On3 NIL Deals, https://www.on3.com/db/emily-cole -162404/.

16   L. S. Fortes, G. P. Berriel, H. Faro, C. G. Freitas-Júnior, and L. A. Peyré-Tartaruga, "Can Prolongate Use of Social Media Immediately Before Training Worsen High Level Male Volleyball Players' Visuomotor Skills?" *Perceptual and Motor Skills* 129, no. 6 (2022): 1790–1803.

17   "Total Compensation By Sport," Opendorse, https://biz.opendorse.com /nil-insights/.

18   "Livvy Dunne," On3 NIL Deals, https://www.on3.com/db/livvy-dunne -162353/.

CHAPTER 12

1   Emma Pallant-Browne (@em_pallant), Instagram, https://www.instagram .com/p/Csoa5cJMuIL/?utm_source=ig_web_copy_link&igsh=MzRlOD BiNWFlZA==.

2   "Brief of over 500 women athletes, the Women's National Basketball Players Association, the National Women's Soccer League Players Association, and Athletes for Impact, who have exercised, relied on, or support the Constitutional right to abortion as amici curiae in support of respondents," Case No. 19-1392 (Supreme Court of the United States), https://reproductiverights.org/wp-content/uploads/2021/09/Athletes-Brief .pdf.

3   E. Guenther, E. Sorensen, and L. Champagne, "Title IX Information Increases Female Collegiate Athletes' Intent to Seek Help," *Journal of Intercollegiate Sport* 16, no. 1 (2023): 54–73. https://doi.org/10.17161/jis .v16i1.15816.

4   Diana Greene Foster, "The Turnaway Study," Scribner 2020.

5   Zara Abrams, "The Facts about Abortion and Mental Health," American Psychological Association, June 22, 2022, https://www.apa.org/monitor /2022/09/news-facts-abortion-mental-health.

6   Diane Chen et al., "Psychosocial Functioning in Transgender Youth after 2 Years of Hormones," *New England Journal of Medicine* 388 (January 19, 2023): 240–50, https://www.nejm.org/doi/full/10.1056/NEJMoa2 206297.

7   Layshia Clarendon (@layshiac), "On Jan 13th at 10am I hugged my wife in front of my surgery building," Instagram post, January 29, 2021, https:// www.instagram.com/p/CKpAwB5hYC8/?utm_source=ig_web_copy_link.

8   "Pregnant and Parenting Student-Athletes," NCAA Gender Equity, http:// s3.amazonaws.com/ncaa.org/documents/2021/1/18/PregnancyToolkit.pdf.

9   Alex Morgan (@alexmorgan13), "Well you shouldn't own a team if you can't (financially) support your players," X (formerly Twitter) post, https://x.com/alexmorgan13/status/1616167424327548928?s=20.

10 Alex Azzez, "Becky Sauerbrunn Opens Up about Freezing Embryos, Ending Stigma," NBC Sports, January 6, 2022, https://www.nbcsports .com/on-her-turf/news/becky-sauerbrunn-opens-up-about-freezing -embryos-ending-stigma.

11 Lindsay Crouse, "Allyson Felix: My Own Nike Story," *New York Times,* May 22, 2019, https://www.nytimes.com/2019/05/22/opinion/allyson -felix-pregnancy-nike.html.

12 Alysia Montaño, "Nike Told Me to Dream Crazy, Until I Wanted a Baby," *New York Times*, May 12, 2019, https://www.nytimes.com/2019/05/12 /opinion/nike-maternity-leave.html.

13   Serena Williams (@serenawilliams), "Last week was not easy for me,"
     Instagram post, August 6, 2018, https://www.instagram.com/p/BmJ3
     KMzFRZw/?utm_source=ig_web_copy_link.
14   &Mother, andmother.org, https://andmother.org/.

CHAPTER 13

1   Dawne Vogt, "Research on Women, Trauma, and PTSD," National Center
    for Post-Traumatic Stress Disorder, https://www.ptsd.va.gov/professional
    /treat/specific/ptsd_research_women.asp.
2   Miranda Olff, "Sex and Gender Differences in Post-Traumatic Stress
    Disorder: An Update," *European Journal of Psychotraumatology* 8, no. 4.
    https://www.tandfonline.com/doi/abs/10.1080/20008198.2017.1351204.
3   Angela J. Hattery, Earl Smith, Katelyn Foltz, and Marissa Kiss, "Ineffective
    Policies for Gender-Based Violence in Sports Result in a Lack of
    Accountability," Brookings, April 4, 2023, https://www.brookings.edu
    /articles/ineffective-policies-for-gender-based-violence-in-sports-result-in
    -lack-of-accountability/.
4   J. J. Freyd, "What is a Betrayal Trauma? What is Betrayal Trauma Theory?"
    Retrieved September 21, 2023, http://pages.uoregon.edu/dynamic/jjf
    /defineBT.html.
5   National Center for PTSD, "Self-Help and Coping," https://www.ptsd.va
    .gov/gethelp/selfhelp_coping.asp.
6   "How to Cope with Traumatic Stress," American Psychological Association,
    https://www.apa.org/topics/trauma/stress.

CHAPTER 14

1   Serena Williams (@serenawilliams), Instagram, August 22, 2023, https://
    www.instagram.com/p/CwQl-n9PJjx/?utm_source=ig_web_copy_link.
2   A. Odone et al., "Italian Working Group on Retirement and Health. Does
    Retirement Trigger Depressive Symptoms? A Systematic Review and
    Meta-Analysis," *Epidemiology and Psychiatry Science* 1 (December 2021):
    30:e77. doi: 10.1017/S2045796021000627.

CONCLUSION

1   "We Are Angel City," HBO, 2023, https://www.hbo.com/angel-city.

INDEX

ABOUT THE AUTHORS

KATIE STEELE

Katie Steele is a licensed marriage and family therapist and cofounder of Thrive Mental Health, an outpatient mental health clinic in Bend, Oregon. She is also the founder of Athlete's Mental Health Foundation, a 501(c)(3) launched in January 2023. Competing in track and cross-country at the University of Oregon and Florida State University, Katie placed second team all PAC-10 as a redshirt freshman. Through her experiences as an NCAA Division-I athlete, Katie has developed a mission to help integrate mental health care into athletics. Her three kids help fuel her passion to ensure healthy sports systems for all and that children are afforded opportunities to cultivate a lifelong love of physical activity.

TIFFANY BROWN

Dr. Tiffany Brown is a faculty member at the University of Oregon in the couples and family therapy graduate program and a licensed marriage and family therapist. She received her doctoral degree in marriage and family therapy from Texas Tech University. Clinically, Dr. Brown works with people dealing with self-harm, trauma, grief, and issues of substance use and recovery. For many years, Dr. Brown has served as a mentor in the University of Oregon's mentor program for athletes, served as a consultant and teacher to the University of Oregon athletics program regarding mental health, and has worked clinically with student athletes. Professionally, she balances her time between graduate teaching, clinical work, administration, and research. An avid sports fan, she is often found kayaking and on adventures around the Oregon coast.

ERIN STROUT

Erin Strout is a journalist who writes about health, fitness, and Olympic sports with a focus on the issues that women face as they strive to perform and feel their best. Her work has appeared in the *Washington Post*, ESPN, *Self* magazine, *Women's Health*, *Outside*, *Triathlete*, and more. She also served as senior writer at *Women's Running*, contributing editor at *Runner's World*, and senior editor at *Running Times*. Erin coauthored the book *Race Everything: How to Conquer Any Race at Any Distance in Any Environment and Have Fun Doing It*, with Bart Yasso. Since 2013, Erin has covered the top levels of track and field and distance running, from the World Marathon Majors to the Rio and Tokyo Olympics. She is also a former staff reporter for the *Chronicle of Higher Education*, where she covered philanthropy and wrote in-depth pieces concerning the NCAA and campus health. An enthusiastic runner and dog lover, Erin lives and plays in Flagstaff, Arizona.